DETOX
Yourself

DETOX
Yourself

JANE SCRIVNER

piatkus

PIATKUS

First published in Great Britain in 1998 by Piatkus Books
This paperback edition published in 2007 by Piatkus Books
This edition published in 2007
Reprinted 2008, 2009, 2010, 2011, 2012

A CIP catalogue record for this book
is available from the British Library.

ISBN 978-0-7499-2828-5

Typeset by Action Publishing Technology Ltd, Gloucester
Printed and bound in Great Britain by
Clays Ltd, St Ives plc

Papers used by Piatkus are from well-managed forests
and other responsible sources.

MIX
Paper from
responsible sources
FSC® C104740

Piatkus
An imprint of
Little, Brown Book Group
100 Victoria Embankment
London EC4Y 0DY

An Hachette UK Company
www.hachette.co.uk

www.piatkus.co.uk

Contents

Introduction

Detox is not about giving everything up for a month. It's not about staying in and hibernating because it is impossible to live a normal life while following a detox programme, and it's not about being miserable for 30 days.

Detox is about making small changes and different choices – and getting huge results.

We all eat every day; detox just changes what we eat. We all shop for food; detox just makes us buy different things. We all want more energy to do more things; detox gives us bags more energy, a positive mood and a way forward that is simple, effective and easy to follow. We just have to invest a bit of time in getting used to it.

Detox is suitable for everyone. The only thing stopping you from being successful on a detox programme is your attitude. Whatever your job, whatever hours you keep, however many children you have, there really is no reason why you cannot detox: it is, after all, just healthy eating.

I wrote the first version of *Detox Yourself* in 1998 because I recognised that we don't give our bodies the food we need to fuel the lifestyle we want. Since then, the response has been phenomenal; the feedback, amazingly positive – and the results speak for themselves. Anyone who has followed the programme completely has been rewarded for their efforts. Getting flexible with their food choices has helped them to discover a whole new world. They lose weight, look great, have a positive attitude and bags of energy.

Quite rightly we want to live life to the full. We want to do everything and be everything to everyone. The only problem is that we think our bodies can do this without our help. In fact, we expect our bodies to do it in spite of ourselves.

We start the day with caffeine, because we think we cannot live without it – mistake number one. We skip breakfast because we are too busy to eat – mistake number two. We rush a sandwich down at lunch and then snack on chocolate mid-afternoon because we don't have time to eat or prepare a proper lunch – mistake number three, and then we relax in the evening with a large glass of alcohol (or two) and a takeaway meal.

We then expect to get up the next morning and do it all again, stress-free and firing on all cylinders. It works for a while but eventually your body just doesn't deliver. And that's where we are now; expecting our bodies to perform and refusing to believe we are responsible for it when they don't. We get tired and moody, we cannot be bothered to do anything properly, but we vow we will do it all better tomorrow.

Well, tomorrow is today: the first day you do a deal with yourself to make some changes that will give you more energy to do more with your day – and with your life. You are going to incorporate some exercise into your day, make different food choices and enjoy some detox treatments. Simple? You bet. You are going to give up caffeine, alcohol, wheat, dairy, preservatives and additives – for just 30 days. You will see how fabulous you feel for relatively little effort and then you can decide what to reintroduce and what to leave out. It's your choice: I will show you the way, but you take the steps.

We are detoxing your diet and your attitudes to food and your body. Detox gives you the good habits to live your life to the full. It really is that simple … go on, I dare you.

PART 1

Before you Begin

1

Why Detox?

'I feel completely turned around and won't be turning back.'

Linda, Guildford

'After 30 days on detox I felt fabulous. Everyone commented on how great I looked, which was confirmation that it really worked. It was so much easier to do than I originally thought – I'm going to carry on!'

Ms Anderson, Hemel Hempstead

WHY SHOULD YOU DETOX?

Two more hours per day, glowing skin, weight loss of several pounds, high energy levels, clear-headedness, higher thresholds for stress and tension, no cellulite, good body tone and a great feeling of being relaxed and totally in control of how you feel – that's why you should detox.

Ten years of experience; ten years of people following the programme and getting the results they want. Some say they have more energy, some say they are more able to cope with anything that is thrown at them, and some say they lose weight and feel fab. Whatever the reason, it seems doing this detox gets you where you want to be, mentally, physically and emotionally.

The proof is in the pudding – well, perhaps the grilled pineapple with flaked almond crunch! Yes, it's been ten years since I wrote *Detox Yourself* and it's time to make some subtle changes to incorporate what I have learned, how the world of detox has changed and the new thinking about healthy eating.

I used to say that we know how to eat healthily, but we just don't. Now the thinking is that we *don't* actually know how to eat healthily and we don't know when to stop eating once our bodies have had enough. We eat socially, we eat because we are hungry, we eat because it's delicious and we eat simply because we want to eat.

We used to eat to survive. We ate, felt satiated and we stopped eating. Food was scarce and fairly basic: meat, berries and plants – not quite the stuff the Michelin stars are made of. Now there is a limitless selection of food available to us. However, the human body is remarkable in that we can feed it almost anything and it will absorb the goodness and expel the badness. It's the most efficient waste-disposal system we know – the most efficient detox system we know.

The problem we have created is that we tend to feed the body more of the foods that it cannot use and less of the nourishing foods that it needs to work efficiently. It then has to spend more time sorting and expelling waste. If we continue to feed it foods that it cannot use or tolerate, it realises that it is fighting a losing battle and then begins to compromise or compensate and tries to carry on despite what we feed it. If our bodies are always compensating then we are never going to feel 100 per cent.

The Detox Programme is designed to stop the body having to settle for second best. It makes sure that the foods you eat for the 30 days are good, wholesome foods, which are eaten primarily to nourish, replenish and regenerate the body.

Victims of our own success

As human beings, we have evolved steadily in response to our bodies' needs in order to survive. Over thousands of years we have become more sophisticated, in all areas of our lives. The way we live our lives has changed, and, with that, technology has advanced rapidly to meet new demands. Food technology is part of that advance. We source, refine and process many foodstuffs that were not available to us until relatively recently. Caveman ate berries and plants, and caught meat and fish. Modern man has pre-packed, pre-peeled and ready-mixed – progress indeed!

Also, the 'modern' way of doing things means we don't do things in moderation. We are time-poor; we need to pack twice as much into every day and we have devised short cuts to enable this to happen. This, in turn, means that our meals and the way we regard food has changed, so our food is also subjected to many short cuts.

Ultimately, something has to give. If we want to do more, get more out of life, be more successful, achieve more and be more satisfied, the very thing that can make this happen – a healthy body, full of energy and fighting fit – is the first thing we ignore. We eat on the run, we skip meals, we snack and drink too much, we use stimulants such as tea and coffee and we use relaxants like alcohol, we use energy boosters like chocolate and sugar. Anything that would actually feed us and keep us going, we perceive to be time-consuming and inconvenient.

Well, the inconvenient truth is that good food is good for you. No matter which way you cut it, you will be healthier with a healthy diet. If you cut out the foods that do not feed your body and feed your body with the ones that do, you will never look back.

Following a detox programme will give you the tools to make your life healthier and happier – over 150,000 readers cannot be wrong.

WHAT DOES DETOX ACTUALLY DO?

Detoxing is what our bodies do all day long; it's what they were designed to do. We just overload the systems with what we feed our bodies. Following an active detox programme will stop the overload, show us how we feel when we eat the right foods and enable us to learn which foods work for us.

The media devote a lot of column inches and sound bites to telling us that detoxing does not work, that we are not full of toxins and poisons and that detoxing is not good for you or it's a waste of time.

The truth is, I don't believe that anyone who writes about detox, and there are many, is trying to say that we are full of toxins and that the foods we eat are poisoning us. What I personally *am* trying to say is that we eat a lot of the wrong foods: foods that are of no use to us, foods that the body needs time to process but that provide no nutritional value, foods that are wasting our bodies' time and energy. Time and energy that we could well use to live our lives to the full.

The definition of 'toxin' is 'poison' and the word 'poison' is defined as a 'substance that, when introduced into or absorbed by a living organism (that's you and me), may destroy life or injure health'. In removing the foods from our diet that are hard work for the body, that have no nutritional value and that 'injure health', we will be left with a good, balanced, nutritional diet. We will be eating the foods our bodies can use – nobody can argue that one.

The advantages of following the Detox Programme:

- It will give you control over your life again and bring the natural balance back into your body, thus helping you to achieve your peak of health.

- Everything in the programme is designed to fuel the body and teach it to use its own resources efficiently.

- It provides the body with all the energy it requires to operate normally, as well as more energy to 'mend' any damage already caused.

- It will rid your body of all the side effects of any bad habits, and will instil some ground rules that will mean you can, indeed, do twice as much every day but without putting any unnecessary strain on your health.

- It will cleanse your system.

- It will enhance your circulation and improve your immune system.

- It's the only way to get rid of your cellulite.

How Will It Do This?

The Detox Programme feeds your body with the ultimate combination of foods. By closely following a recommended food list and exercise plan you can bring your body into total balance. After doing this for 30 days, you will have changed the way you eat, changed the food decisions you make, and have learned how you feel when you eat well. You will notice the difference if you don't eat well.

You will have developed good eating habits in place of your previous bad habits because it takes a minimum of 21 days to form a habit – good or bad. The programme lasts for 30 days for a reason, not because I'm mean but because I know that if you can do 30 days you will have picked up some good, healthy life habits. The good thing about habits is that you don't even know you are doing them, so it will become really easy to continue being healthy for ever.

Many of the normal, everyday foods we eat can cause problems if we get too much or not enough. More extreme imbalances are well known, for instance, lack of iron causing anaemia, too much alcohol causing addiction, and lack of vitamin C causing scurvy, but few of us are aware that very common foods can have a similar effect if not treated sensibly.

During detox all processed and refined foods are excluded. Everything is eaten in as natural and unprocessed a state as possible, and if it's not possible to do so the items in question are not included. No additives are allowed, and little, if anything, is taken away.

If the food doesn't look like it has just been picked, just dug up or just caught then don't eat it – it's not detox!

In addition to excluding all the 'bad' foods, we include more of the 'good' foods that are often neglected or not recognised as being beneficial. There are many foods that can actively improve a condition or boost the general well-being of an individual which don't readily spring to mind as part of everyday eating, such as:

- Dried fruit

- Raw vegetables

- Garlic

- Sprouted seeds and beans

- Rice cakes

- Hummus

- Beetroot

as well as foods whose value is more commonly understood:

- Fresh fruit

- Fresh vegetables

- Fish

- Herbal teas

- Pulses, such as beans and lentils

- Water

The road to total balance is not, however, followed purely through food and nutrition. With a view to increasing the efficiency of the body's internal systems such as the liver, the kidneys, the circulation and the lymph glands, we will also look at:

- Self-massage techniques

- Dry-skin brushing

- Posture

- Exercise

- Breathing techniques

- Aromatherapy oils

- The many other complementary ways to speed up the detox process.

WILL IT BE DIFFICULT?

To be perfectly honest, at times, yes, it will be difficult. Hey, we are all human beings, so making any change, no matter how small, needs concentration and effort. The human brain likes to play tricks, just as when we resolve to stay on track or eat healthily, the brain starts to draw our attention to the chocolate in the fridge or the crisps in the cupboard. What is more, when we announce we are on a diet or following a detox programme, our fellow human beings hear it as an all-out challenge to make us fail or fall off the wagon.

You owe this kind of programme to yourself. You have to decide that this is what you want. If you keep this positive frame of mind, then the programme will give only benefits and will be easily enjoyed and adhered to. But if you decide that it will be an inconvenience and something that you have to 'shoehorn' into 28 days, then perhaps you should reconsider and give the programme the priority it deserves – postpone it to a more convenient time or make more time now so that it can be accommodated more readily. The Detox Programme is one of the most positive steps you can take and should be treated and enjoyed that way – treat yourself!

You will also see that further on in the programme there are some hints and tips on how to stay on track when you are thinking of throwing the towel in. These suggest ways to motivate yourself to keep going when you really feel like giving up and give some words of encouragement and treats that you can have to stay focused. There are also some suggestions on how to get back on track or back on the wagon if you have inadvertently fallen off. I have even included some 'illegal snacks' for those human moments of madness – I've been there.

HOW LONG DOES IT LAST?

Detoxing should become a way of life! The first time you follow the programme, it should last a minimum of 30 days, which allows sufficient time to 'spring clean' your body. If you try to do it in less time, the results are not as satisfactory. It is a full 30 days of optimum nutrition and 30 days of developing good habits.

If you then undertake the total Detox Programme on a subsequent occasion you will begin to notice and 'feel' the signs that indicate you have detoxed completely: you are eating the right foods to feed your body back to full fitness. It is likely that this time around it will take less than the initial 30 days.

Ideally, as you start to reach the end of your 30-day programme you will start to decide which elements you will keep and which elements you will discontinue. Parts of the programme will stay with you for ever, and other parts will not be tried again.

It is likely that you will be about to embark on a very different way of eating, and elements of this will stay with you for the rest of your life. Foods that you enjoyed before the programme may not seem so enjoyable afterwards; this is generally due to their levels of toxins. Coffee is quite difficult to give up, but once you have spent 30 days without it, it is likely that the flavour will have become too strong or too processed for your newly revived palate. Similarly, foods that you might previously not have considered, such as rice cakes and fresh fish, will become a staple part of your eating plan.

There will also be times when you think that you may have overdone the high living and rich foods and feel like a one-week detox just to give your body a chance to recover some energy. Once you have completed the initial 30-day programme it is entirely up to you to choose how to use the programme and tailor it to fit your lifestyle.

HOW DO YOU FEEL?

Where do I start? Fresher, healthier, happier, more in control, self-satisfied, like you have achieved something really important, full of energy, more positive, clearer skin and sparkling eyes. Wave goodbye to mood swings and to feeling starving one minute and bloated the next. You will be better company – as long as you don't become a detox bore! You may feel more confident in yourself, and as you look fabulous and feel fitter you will have the confidence to try different things or even make some major changes. You will have a clearer head and a clear idea of how to feed your body so that it works for you.

Ultimately you will feel wonderful, as if you have much more energy at both ends of the day. When you wake up in the morning you may not wish to jump out of bed, but you won't feel lethargic or as if you need more sleep. You will be tired when you go to bed, but the feeling of exhaustion won't be there any more. You will sleep soundly and will wake less during the night. You will feel more vital.

You may experience some side effects, but these really depend on how you lived prior to following the programme. If you were a heavy tea or coffee drinker you may experience one or two days of mild headaches as your body 'comes off' the caffeine. You have taught your body how to expect these stimulants and now it needs to learn to live without them. Similarly, heavy sugar eaters, or heavy bread and pasta consumers, may experience a temporary energy loss as the body adjusts to the programme.

More general effects may be a small outbreak of spots – not generally on the face. These show that the body is cleansing itself of all toxins; since the skin is the largest organ of the body it is the most obvious area for elimination and cleansing. A furry tongue is common in the early days but this will clear. Halitosis (bad breath) can also occur – again, only for a short time. All these symptoms indicate that the detox is working and there are ways to make the transition less painful for you and for others.

Other side effects are generally due to misinterpreting the programme. For instance there may be occasions when you will feel tired, which probably means that you are not eating enough of the essential foods. These areas are covered fully in the relevant sections and more so in the troubleshooting checklist at the end of Chapter 4.

All the expected side effects are positive indications that the programme is cleaning out your body and giving all your internal systems the valuable vitamins, minerals and nutrients they need to work at peak levels.

If any of the side effects persist for more than a couple of days, then you do need to visit the checklist; you are doing something wrong and you need to change it. Detoxing should be good for you, with only a few 'changeover blips' as your body gets used to good foods – not a hard task to be endured.

How Do I Start?

Before you start, plan, plan, plan. Once you have decided to reward yourself with a new, revitalised, detoxed you, then read on. The following pages tell you everything you need to know and do prior to starting the programme, give you a step-by-step guide during the programme and then offer plenty of ideas about how to maintain the programme once you have completed your initial 30 days.

If you plan your programme, prepare the right foods and stock your house with 'detox stuff', then you will find it much easier to complete it successfully. Simply waking one morning and deciding 'today's the day!', will be much harder on you as you open the fridge where the star attraction is the leftover takeaway and there is no detox alternative.

Fail to plan and you plan to fail. This is one of those nauseating phrases I learned in my days in advertising but I have to say, unfortunately, it is very, very true.

So, let's make plans ...

2

How the Body Functions

Before starting the Detox Programme it is worth knowing how the body operates and how it will respond to detoxing. What causes the 'tox' to be there in the first place? What gets detoxed? And why does the body need our help – why doesn't it do the job itself?

First we need to look at the internal systems that will carry out your internal detox, and at what exactly makes up or causes the waste and toxins we are talking about. Only when you have understood these concepts and processes should you embark on the programme itself.

The human body is a highly sophisticated structure of organs and systems formulated to achieve balance and harmony. It uses foods and fluids for nourishment, repair and maintenance – what is known as metabolism. Our systems and organs process these foods, keep what they need and eliminate the waste – so, yes, the body does detox itself quite naturally. It is when we upset this balance, causing an overload of waste, that things can start to go wrong. We are giving our bodies too much to do, and we all know how we react if we have too much to do: things go wrong, slow down and we start operating 'under par'.

The liver, kidneys, lymph system and skin are all critical to the smooth running of our bodies' natural detoxing process.

THE LIVER

Of the liver's several functions that are vital to health, two concern metabolism and detoxification. The liver takes the poisonous or toxic substances that enter our bodies via food or the environment and converts them to a form that they can use, store safely or eliminate.

THE KIDNEYS

These organs are involved in many essential processes including filtering toxic wastes out of the blood and eliminating them from the body in urine. They are also responsible for maintaining the correct amount of fluid in the body and regulating the balance of potassium and sodium (vital for the correct flow of fluids in the systems).

THE LYMPH SYSTEM

This system acts as a waste disposal facility for the body. Lymph, a liquid produced by lymph glands in various parts of the body, absorbs dead cells, excess fluids and other waste products from foods and takes them to the lymph nodes. Here the waste is filtered and eventually fed into the blood and on to one of the eliminatory organs – skin, liver or kidneys – to be passed out via perspiration, faeces or urine.

THE SKIN

This is the largest organ in the body and serves many vital functions.

A mirror to our health

The skin can be a useful indicator of what is happening within our bodies. 'Looking a bit pale', 'looking well', 'glowing' and 'in the pink' are all everyday phrases used to describe our health through looking at our skin.

The skin mirrors what is happening internally – it is said that the chin area reflects exactly what is happening in the stomach and gut – in other words, it reflects your diet and what you are eating. We have all had an outbreak of nasty spots on our chin at some time or another, and if you think back it will generally relate to an unhealthy period of eating or drinking!

If we are under stress, our skin looks tired and pale. If we are ill, the skin loses colour. If we are severely ill, jaundice (yellowing of the skin), lesions or weeping wounds are just some extreme examples of what can occur.

Excretion

As an organ of elimination the skin is a mere beginner in relation to the liver and kidneys, but it still excretes large quantities of waste products: water, salts, uric acid, ammonia and urea. The skin is like a huge sieve or colander – the goodness stays in and the waste passes out. If the liver and kidneys are overworked or not working efficiently the result may be a skin complaint such as eczema, due to the skin having to deal with more waste than normal.

Protection

The skin protects our bodies in many ways. It forms a physical barrier against 'foreign' substances. It produces an acidic secretion that kills off harmful micro-organisms. It is semi-permeable and regulates what can enter and exit the body. And it prevents excess water loss so as to avoid dehydration.

Body temperature

Our skin regulates our body temperature. If we get hot through exercise or because we are in a hot environment our bodies produce sweat, which cools the skin and our bodies as it evaporates from the surface of the skin. If we get cold, our blood vessels constrict and reduce the flow of blood to the top layers of the skin, thus reducing the loss of heat.

Warning signals

Our skin is our early warning system against danger. If we touch something too hot or too cold, the nerves in our skin send messages to the brain to withdraw or take appropriate action.

THE BODY IN BALANCE

Our long-term health relies on keeping ourselves and our bodies in balance, so that any undue stress or strain that the body experiences can be dealt with efficiently, allowing it to return to normal after a short period of recovery. If any one of the organs or systems described above is not fully functional, things begin to slow down and can eventually result in an overload of waste and toxins.

A body that is out of balance will need considerably longer to recover, as more strain is being put on the systems to process the excess waste and toxins – feelings of sluggishness and lethargy become more frequent. However, if the body is fully fit and healthy the amount of waste matter to be dealt with is at normal levels and this processing is under control, so we feel well and have plenty of energy.

The detox process is designed to keep all these eliminatory organs in tip-top tone and condition – in short, in balance.

The mind

We must also think about the positive changes on our emotions and thoughts when considering a detox programme. The brain supplies us with our emotions and our feelings – our moods. Many people find that they are becoming grouchy or short-tempered for no apparent reason. Well, just as importantly as the major organs in the body, we must not forget the nutrition for our brains. If we eat the wrong types of foods or not enough of the right types, our brains are affected. We have mood swings, serotonin (the feel-good chemical released in our brains) levels are reduced, sugar levels rise and dip making us speed up temporarily and feel more alert, but then the slump that inevitably follows makes us feel more tired than before – at a low on both a physical and mental level.

Our ability to concentrate can also be dictated by diet and hydration, so this is also an important issue.

Suffice to say, every part of our body and mind can be affected positively or negatively by what we eat. We tend to think we are a human being and food is something we do in isolation to make us feel full. We fail to realise that how healthy we are is a side effect of what we eat. It shouldn't be left to chance, it shouldn't be that our bodies have to spend time 'picking out' the good stuff that they can use and discarding the bad stuff, like a treasure hunter going through a skip!

How do we get out of balance?

By living our lives the way we do. There are many ways to throw our body's careful harmony off course, and they all contribute to overloading the eliminatory organs and systems with waste and toxins or slowing them down, both of which can result in their malfunction.

Some forms of waste and toxins occur naturally in the body:

- Every day, through metabolism, the body processes and eliminates billions of worn out and dead cells quite normally.

- The body processes all excess fluid that is no longer required.

- Following illness or injury, the body eliminates dead or scar tissue.

None of these waste product processes should be interfered with, as they are crucial to a normal healthy body. However, there are several areas where we can consciously decrease the introduction of waste into our bodies by:

- Getting fitter, as being unfit can slow down your metabolic rate and so decrease the detox activity within your body.

- Getting well, as being ill will mean that the body functions are disturbed and concentrating on recovery; again this will slow down the internal detox process.

- Eating better, as eating badly or eating only fast foods means the body doesn't get all the necessary nutrients.

- Reducing stress, as being under stress puts the body into fight-or-flight mode (see page 24).

There are also many waste products, toxins and situations that we can and should avoid:

- Cigarettes, alcohol, caffeine and drugs are all products that the body cannot absorb and use and so they add to the mounting levels of waste.

- A diet too high in fats and sugars will add to the waste.

- The environment adds to the waste – pollution, exhaust fumes and pesticides are just some of the culprits.

- Over the past century we have developed the food manufacturing industry in such a way that the number and quantity of additives and preservatives have increased phenomenally in our now more sophisticated and more complicated diet

- We also refine the goodness out of many of the original basic nutritional foodstuffs and hence eat refined wheat, refined flour, refined sugar and so on. Refining foods in this way is sometimes a process more sophisticated than our digestive systems can cope with, so we develop intolerances and the body makes compromises to cope.

Most of us can say that some or all of these are currently a regular part of our diet and lifestyle. This means that we now consume many types of food that the body cannot assimilate and many chemicals that, if not eliminated, will act as toxins in the body. This situation increases the number of food types that the body leaves partially or totally undigested, and so increases the levels of waste that it has to deal with to remain healthy and in balance. The skip holds more waste than treasure!

All this excess waste needs to be sorted and eliminated, but if there is too much for the body to deal with a build-up will result. In high concentrations these waste materials become toxic and can 'poison' the body. In a healthy, fit person the body can assimilate and eliminate all wastes and toxins as and when they occur; there are not too many and they are easy to deal with. In a tired, unhealthy or ill body, the build-up of this waste will start to affect the efficiency of the organs and lead to sluggishness, fatigue and eventually illness. It is this build-up that the Detox Programme will initially decrease and eventually, through new eating habits, erase completely so that our bodies are being given only foods that they can use or eliminate easily and naturally.

STRESS AS A CONTRIBUTING FACTOR

Stress changes the body's normal state, and we need a degree of stress in order to be alert and active to prepare and deal with outside stimuli. Stress causes a natural 'fight-or-flight' reaction in our bodies – we become immediately responsive by either running away or fighting back, and this protects us from danger or difficult situations.

The body reacts to stress by sending a hormone called adrenaline to the legs (to enable us to run away) or to the shoulders and upper torso muscles (to enable us to physically fight the enemy). This was good for our caveman ancestors whose problems were not those of deadlines or traffic jams but those of hunting food or being eaten themselves! They used up all this adrenaline quickly, but when we are put under pressure today we stay in a prolonged state of alertness which, if it continues, will have a damaging effect on our bodies.

At this time of stress the body needs all its resources and so all the other bodily systems temporarily slow down or cease. Blood, for instance, moves away from the digestive system to the muscles in order to prepare for physical action, the bowels empty, the heart rate increases, blood pressure increases, sweating occurs, the pupils dilate, the mouth becomes dry as food is not required. In short, the body has turned away from the essential processes of digestion and absorption of foods and nutrients for repair and maintenance in favour of self-defence.

Remaining in a prolonged state of stress will result in undigested food, the secreting of toxins by the body and slow and inefficient processing of the waste products in the body. All this causes excess and overload which, if not dealt with quickly, will simply build up each time the body is subjected to further stress.

Part of the Detox Programme involves getting rid of, or at least managing, some of the stress in our lives in order to minimise the unnecessary disturbance to our bodies.

What physically happens when there is a build-up or overload of waste, toxins and stress?

The human body is very sophisticated and will still function well under some extremely adverse conditions. The build-up of stress, waste and toxins happens very gradually and the body will adapt to these new conditions. But each time it is required to adapt, some of the efficiency is lost. Eventually we start to get warning signs that it is time to implement some changes ourselves before irreversible damage is caused.

The overload of toxins in the system will generally result in a feeling of fatigue, both physically and mentally. This is caused by each of the eliminatory organs or systems having its own problems as a build-up of waste occurs, with each organ or system reacting differently. Below are some of the more obvious effects that are pertinent to the Detox Programme.

Extended periods of stress will cause extended periods of poor nutrition, bad absorption, increased blood pressure and heart rate, and inefficient functioning of the bodily systems. Nutrition, repair and maintenance soon become replaced with basic survival, and the internal eliminatory organs become sluggish in their processing of undigested foods and waste. As the body deals with stress we feel exhausted and mentally drained.

The liver takes potentially damaging substances that we have introduced into our daily routines, such as alcohol, drugs, poisons and caffeine, and breaks them down into forms that can be eliminated via the faeces and urine. The liver also takes toxic substances produced by the body and removes them by elimination to prevent self-poisoning. If the liver becomes overworked and inefficient, illnesses such as jaundice and gallstones can occur.

If the blood contains too many toxins and waste products the kidneys will have to work harder than usual, and if we don't take optimum care of these organs this may lead to their sluggish or inefficient functioning. If any of these functions fail, serious illness will result. In the same way, if any of these functions cause the kidneys to be overworked the result can be tiredness and lethargy.

Poor lymph drainage due to excess waste results in a build-up of fluid containing waste products. As we know, this waste can become toxic and stagnant and eventually will induce feelings of bloating and fatigue. In addition, tissue can be damaged due to the excess fluid.

How do we prevent this build-up or overload of waste and toxins?

It is likely, if you are reading this book, that you feel you have already got a certain build-up of toxins. You may not be aware of any actual feelings of illness, but you may have some side effects of a gradual build-up: tiredness, lethargy, irritable bowel, mouth ulcers, spots and blemishes, dull complexion, low energy levels, bloated feelings, fluid retention, muscle fatigue, heavy periods or headaches.

Avoiding the causes of waste is not always easy, but by following a carefully planned eating programme and being aware of your environment and surroundings you can greatly reduce them. A formalised detoxification programme will not only provide the body with unprocessed, pure foods but also concentrate on specific foods that will actively create the ideal environment for your body to regain its natural balance. Such a programme will also cover all complementary activities that enhance the food aspects: stress reduction and management, exfoliation, breathing, massage, additional treatments, self-treatment, exercise and so on. Once you have eliminated all toxins from your diet and hence your body, you will be in a much better position to maintain this status and keep the balance.

Now that you have a basic understanding of how the body functions, of what wastes and toxins are, how they affect our bodies and what we can do to avoid them, you are ready to start!

3

Preparing for Detox

BEFORE COMMENCING THE PROGRAMME

The Detox Programme is about eating a healthy balanced diet. You will be eating a minimum of three meals a day and should not feel starved. Healthy eating is not dangerous and is positively encouraged for everyone. However, for some people with certain conditions, the changes required in your current diet may be a little too much for your body to handle all at once. There are very few reasons why you should not start the Detox Programme without medical advice, but where they exist, these reasons are very important indeed and should always be taken into consideration. You should not start the programme without medical advice if any of the following applies to you at the time of your detox:

• You are pregnant

• You are breastfeeding

• You are undergoing medical treatment for any illness or condition

• You are recovering from a serious illness

• You are taking any prescribed or recreational drugs

• You have any doubts about your own medical health

Always consult your doctor if you are in any doubt as to whether this programme is suitable for you.

How to Plan the 30 Days

When you have decided that you want to detox, the first thing to work out is how much of a change from your normal way of eating it is going to be. Doing a short self-assessment will enable you to see if there are some extra things that you might want to start a few weeks in advance of the programme itself. Doing so may make the programme less of a shock to the system and, therefore, ultimately easier and more enjoyable. If you complete the following self-assessment you can work out the best way to start your own detox and the best time to schedule it. Circle or tick the choices below that best describe your current situation.

Self-assessment

How do you rate your current diet?
(Score 3) Very healthy
(Score 2) Fairly healthy
(Score 1) Bad

How are your energy levels?
(Score 3) Good
(Score 2) OK
(Score 1) Low

Which best describes your activity levels?
(Score 3) Regular exercise and/or an active job or life
(Score 2) Some exercise but a sedentary job
(Score 1) No exercise and a sedentary job

How much water do you drink per day?
(Score 3) 1.7 litres (3 pints)
(Score 2) 3–4 glasses
(Score 1) Fewer than 3 glasses

How much coffee and tea do you drink per day?
(Score 3) Few/none
(Score 2) About 3 cups
(Score 1) About 6 cups or more

How much alcohol do you drink per week? (one unit
equals a medium glass of wine, half a pint of beer or
lager, or one measure of spirits)
(Score 3) 0–6 units
(Score 2) 8–12 units
(Score 1) 15 units or more

**How much fresh fruit or vegetables do you eat every
day?**
(Score 3) 3–4 portions
(Score 2) 1–2 portions
(Score 1) 1 or none

How often do you eat take-away food?
(Score 3) Less than once a week
(Score 2) Once a week
(Score 1) 3–4 times a week

How many carbonated drinks do you have per day (cola/fruit flavoured drinks and so on)?
(Score 3) Less than one a day
(Score 2) One a day
(Score 1) More than one a day

How often do you use salt?
(Score 3) Add to food occasionally
(Score 2) Add to food after tasting
(Score 1) Add to cooking and also to food without tasting

Now add your scores together and interpret them as follows:

Scores 15 or above

If you have scored 15 or above in the self-assessment you should be able to start the Detox Programme on Day 1 as described, without any further preparation.

Scores below 15

If you have scored below 15 in the self-assessment you should consider making some changes before you embark on Day 1. In the month before detox consider changing your daily life along these lines:

- Start doing some mild exercise, such as a walk at lunchtime or running up and down the stairs five times before bed – anything that will increase your pulse rate for 20 minutes each day.

- Make sure you drink at least 1 litre (1³/4 pints) of water a day.

- Reduce your alcohol intake by half.

- Reduce your intake of coffee, tea and fizzy drinks by half.

- Make sure you eat at least three portions of fruit and three portions of vegetables each day. A portion of fruit is an apple or a pear and so on, and a portion of vegetables is one large serving spoon or more.

- Limit take-away food to once a month.

WHEN TO START

When you have completed the self-assessment above you can see if you are cleared for take-off, or if you need to revise your current diet before commencing. Whatever your results, ideally, you need to allocate your 30 days well in advance. There is no really bad time of year to detox, just perhaps a more convenient time for you personally. The early part of the year is often a good time – once you have recovered after Christmas the next few months are a time for taking stock, making life decisions and saving money! Depending on when Easter falls, February or March can be good candidates. There are plenty of fruit and vegetables around and the spring and summer social occasions – summer barbecues, children's parties and so on – have not yet started, they are weekends away. Having said that, summer could be a good time for you if you are the kind of person who loves salads and fresh fish.

The main consideration is to try to find a start time

when you have relatively few social commitments. Beginning the programme on the weekend of your best friend's wedding is likely to push your self-control to its limits, and turning up with a Tupperware container full of rice and veggies may prove a subject for discussion but will ultimately ruin the day!

There is no need to take time off work. But again, if you know that you have a run of meetings or conferences coming up and there will be caterers' food, this is something to avoid.

If your child's birthday party is on the horizon or if you are hosting the local coffee morning, think twice about starting the programme. This is not because the programme is hard to keep to, but it is a departure from your normal lifestyle and you will make extra work for yourself if you spend most of the time avoiding or adapting to fit these occasions.

In my view, the best day to start is a Sunday or Monday. Plan to have a relatively quiet time socially for the next week or so and don't make any social arrangements in the first week. Thereafter, try to see only close friends and entertain at home or in non fast-food restaurants – you can easily entertain friends without them ever knowing that they are detoxing for the evening. (Chapter 5 is full of useful recipes for such occasions.) Once you have got into the swing of the programme you will be able to plan the remaining days to suit yourself. By the end of the first week you will be much more aware and much less obsessed about what you should be eating, and you will have found a routine for the other activities.

MENTAL PREPARATION

The time when you detox is a time you should enjoy – you deserve to find time for yourself, and you should look upon the Detox Programme as a treat for yourself and your body. Don't think that there are lots of things that you can't have, but that there are lots of things you can. There will be new foods for you to try, lots of ways that you can pamper your body, lots of excuses to book in for treatments, lots of ways to reduce or manage stress, tools to get rid of cellulite and a chance to feel much healthier and much more vital.

So think of the Detox Programme as your own personal month at a health farm – you will be creating your own 'detox oasis'. Enjoy each day of the programme. Don't always think about how long you have to go, but think about how much you have already done and how good you feel. When you tell people what you are doing they will be very interested. Don't tell them how different it is from normal and how time-consuming it is to get everything done, but tell them how many positive changes you have made and how you are doing much more every day due to your increased energy levels. Keep yourself busy, certainly in the early days. When you have eaten in the evening, sitting around wondering what else you can eat can be really disheartening. If you are still hungry, have a little more, or eat slowly – it takes 20 minutes for your mind to tell your body that it's full. I am very aware of how, when temptation or boredom gets in the way, your mind plays tricks on you, tricks like, 'No one will know if I eat his chocolate', 'If I just have one glass of wine it can't harm the programme' or 'I really feel like a coffee and brownie.' I know because I've been there! But let me assure you, if you give in you will be disappointed and if you give in you won't get the results intended. Disappointment will be a shame given how much effort you will be putting in. Do it properly, get the benefits and feel hugely pleased with yourself. Adopting a positive state of mind from the start will make the programme much more satisfying – 'getting through' the programme will make it feel like a struggle and you are more likely to give up or leave the programme incomplete.

PHYSICAL PREPARATION

Although you should be able to follow the programme quite normally without having to buy or use any special equipment, there are some things that you need to gather together or source. Many of these you will already have or will know where to get hold of, but you should do this in plenty of time. Having them ready when you start makes the programme go smoothly; a little preparation is, in any case, never a bad thing and certainly a good habit to get into.

Checklist of essentials

- **Airtight food containers**   A variety of sizes is useful as you can store large amounts (rice and so on) or carry small snacks for when you are on the move.

- **Steamer – metal or bamboo**

  The type you put over or in a pan of hot water to steam vegetables or fish.

- **Skin brush – natural bristles**

  Bristles should be firm but not too stiff, otherwise they may irritate the flesh. You could treat yourself to a Jane Scrivner Detox Brush Bag (see page 202).

- **Exfoliating creams or salt**

  Use up any odds and ends of creams to save money. If they are not exfoliants add a teaspoon of salt or sand and this will do the job, or go to page 202 for details of the Jane Scrivner Detox product range.

- **Loofah or flannel mitt**

  Towelling or natural fibre.

- **Moisturising creams**

  Anything you have at home – take the opportunity to use up all the old bottles of moisturiser that have been hanging around and you haven't thrown away yet.

- **Massage creams or oils**

  Any natural oils are suitable. If you have massage oils these are fine, but sunflower, olive or grapeseed oils from the supermarket or your kitchen cupboards are all great. They are better than cosmetic creams because, being natural products, they

will be completely absorbed
into the skin. See also page
209.

- **Somewhere to exercise**

  Gym, bedroom, stairs,
  lounge, and so on.

- **Bath or shower**

  Daily access to both a bath and
  a shower is ideal, but one or
  the other is fine.

Checklist of optionals/luxuries

- **Sauna or steam room**

  See if there is one in your local
  leisure centre. It will be cheaper
  than a health club and using it
  can be combined with a swim.

- **Juicer**

  This is an absolute luxury, but
  what better time to try than
  during the detox?

- **Weekend or day trip to
  the sea or countryside**

  Breathing fresh air is one of the
  best things for the Detox
  Programme – time away
  is always beneficial.

- **Organic foods**

  There are many suppliers of
  organic fruit, veg and fish
  prepared to supply nationally.
  Using organic foods will
  guarantee that all pesticides are
  eliminated before you even
  start. Organic foods are not
  essential – the fact that you are
  going to be eating fresh foods
  over the next month is
  probably enough of a change.
  But if fruit and vegetables

already form the basis of your
diet then try organics and see
if you notice a difference.

The following topics will be discussed at length in
Chapter 9, but it may be worth sourcing them before you
start. There is a list of contact numbers on page 236
which should help you to find practitioners in your area.

- **Massage, aromatherapy**

  You may be able to find these
  detox treatments locally or,
  even better, some practitioners
  will do home visits.

- **Colonic irrigation**

  Your local health centre should
  be able to help you locate local
  practitioners.

- **Reflexology**

  Again, your local health centre
  or even health food shop may
  be able to give you names of
  local practitioners.

- **LaStone Therapy**

  Find a local practitioner on
  www.lastonetherapy.co.uk
  for an extra-special detox
  acceleration.

There are some more unusual items – on top of your
meals – that you will be required to eat or drink every day,
and these should be bought in advance as you are unlikely
to have them in stock. They are listed here merely for
shopping purposes, and will be fully explained in Chapter
4. Some may sound a bit odd, but all will be revealed later!

Essential shopping

- **Vegetable juices – carrot or beetroot**

  Bottled juice is usually available from health food shops. Start with one bottle. Alternatively, if you have a juicer buy fresh vegetables and juice your own.

- **Olive oil**

  Try to buy extra virgin, cold pressed or first pressed oils as these are purer and contain the highest nutrients. They are available in all supermarkets. 1 litre (2 pints) will do to start.

- **Fresh garlic**

  To start, buy a large bulb so that you can eat one clove a day, if required.

- **Honey**

  Buy one pot, preferably from someone who stocks or produces good-quality, home-produced honey. Manuka grade is probably the best honey available and the most effective.

- **Fresh lemons**

  From greengrocers or supermarkets. Buy three to start.

- **Sprouted beans**

  From health food shops, or buy a sprouter and do your own. You can also sprout your own beans on absorbent paper: simply dampen the paper, sprinkle the seeds over it and leave in a light, sunny place.

Make sure the paper doesn't dry and the beans will sprout in a few days. Mung beans, chick peas and alfalfa are all good. If you cannot find these, replace them with a daily supplement of alfalfa pills.

• **Water**

Filtered or bottled. Still is preferable to fizzy, which can be saved for evenings out. You will need enough for 1.5 litres (2¾ pints) for the first three days. Use tap water if there is no other kind available, or if you live in an area that has good water.

You can gather these items together in preparation for Day 1, but the bulk of the foodstuffs should be bought as and when you would normally do your shopping. The fresher the foods, the more nutrients you will get. Fresh, crisp vegetables will leave you feeling fresh and crisp yourself; old, limp, shrivelled vegetables ... need I say more?

WHAT IT COSTS

If you don't have some or all of the 'essential items' try to borrow them from friends to keep costs down. But if you do buy, these won't be wasted purchases as you will probably continue to use them long after the programme is over. A steamer, plastic containers and skin brushes or flannels should, together, cost less than a good facial –

which you will not need as the detox will leave your skin radiant and pure.

The essential food extras such as vegetable juice and olive oil may mean spending up front, but you will recoup the money during the programme as your fresh foods will cost less than the processed foods that you would normally buy.

This is a great time to find your local markets, local suppliers of produce and local fishmongers rather than huge supermarkets. Know where your food comes from. If you live in the countryside, go to farmers' markets. Really try to buy fruit and veg that come from nearby or, at the very least, the UK (or your own country if you are reading this abroad). Eat seasonally: strawberries in November may have been through a heck of a lot before they get to your kitchen table; we don't want stressed food, we want happy food. We all know how we feel after a long wait at the airport to check in, an even longer flight and then a lengthy wait to get through baggage control – imagine the state of a poor vegetable after all that. Go local, stay fresh and vital.

PART 2

Time to Detox

4

The Detox Programme

'The diet looked pretty daunting, but I found it quite easy
to follow and actually enjoyed it. As well as following the
food programme, I had to use a body brush, shower in
cold water every morning, have massages and take exercise. The results were great. I lost half a stone in the first
three weeks and definitely noticed a reduction in my
cellulite. It's hard work, but I would do it again – it has
been an education.'

Jane, London

Make sure you read this section several times. There will
always be things on the lists that you will forget or
combinations that you do not realise at first, and reading
several times before and during the programme will
ensure that you don't miss any of these. There is a checklist at the end of this chapter for you to use every day. If
reading in detail is not your thing, then make a list of the
types of foods you think are healthy, or you want to eat on
the programme and then go through the food lists to
check whether they are allowed, making sure *all* the ingredients are included in my lists not just half of them!

The Detox Programme is a 'total body experience'. The

approach is holistic and works on every part of the body – internal and external:

- There are foods that are highly nutritional and for that reason I am calling them 'superfoods', and as such a huge portion of them should be included in the programme every day – do not miss these out.

- There are body-care routines that should be followed every day – again, do not miss these out. Either DIY or splash out and book yourself in to have someone else do the work for you – you deserve it.

FOODS ON THE DETOX PROGRAMME

The Detox Programme is very specific: if the foods are not listed in the next few pages, they are not included in the programme. You do not need to be a whizz in the kitchen, but do try to be as varied as possible in your food choices as this will make the programme more interesting. In the same way that you probably follow a routine in your meals at the moment – for instance, toast and coffee for breakfast, sandwiches for lunch and a pasta dish for supper – it is completely normal to fall into a routine of having a similar thing each lunchtime and so on while you are on the programme, just try to make the ingredients slightly different each day. We shall be looking at:

- Superfoods you must have every day and why.

- Everything you can eat for the full 30 days, by category.

- Foods you think would be included but are most definitely not, and why.

Starting the Detox Programme

When you start the programme, from Day 1 to Day 30 you must:

- Drink a cup of hot water and lemon juice first thing every morning.

- During the day drink at least 1.5 litres (2³/₄ pints) of water.

- Include at least one superfood per meal – either as an additional snack or included in the recipe.

- If you scored below 15 on the self-assessment on page 29, take multivitamin supplements every day for the first 15 days.

- Eat at least three meals every day from the food lists, or preferably five slightly smaller meals a day.

- Have at least one portion of rice every day – make sure it is wild, short grain or organic brown rice.

- Have at least three portions of vegetables – one should be raw, juices are aceptable for one portion.

- Have at least three portions of raw fruit, dried fruit can be substituted for one portion.

- Have at least three portions of salad.

- Have at least one portion of non-dairy yogurt, cheese or milk every day. (Non-dairy means goat's or sheep's products, rice products (that is, rice milk) or soya products (that is, soya milk).)

• Have two portions every day of any of the following; pulses, nuts, herbs, olive or any seed oil, or fish.

Keep your food intake balanced and check you are not having the same for every meal – variety is the spice of detox life.

Why you need these foods and this regime

Hot lemon water   The biggest organ of detox is the liver, and starting the day with a squeeze of fresh lemon juice in a cup of hot water will not only refresh and revitalise you but will also clean your palate and 'jump-start' your liver. The lemon is acidic, but is alkaline-forming in the stomach and gut, which is why any pills you take for antacid or cystitis are normally lemon flavoured. This will help to balance the pH in your system during detox. People in many Eastern cultures scrape the surface of their tongue first thing in the morning in the belief that doing so greatly reduces the amount of infections and germs that they carry. You may want to try this, but if not swill the first mouthful of lemon water and spit it out before drinking the rest as normal. Cider vinegar can be substituted, but may be a little sharp for most palates.

Water   Around 80 per cent of our bodies consist of water and we need to drink 1.5 litres minimum per day to keep that level stable. In hot weather or during exercise you should increase this amount to cover the deficit. Water replenishes, cleanses, rejuvenates and restores, and is probably the most important single item in the Detox Programme. At first, the essential 1.5 litres (2³/₄ pints) may feel too much, and you will spend a lot of time going to the bathroom! Changing your eating habits to include the foods recommended on the programme will also increase your water intake, as many healthy foods are high in water content. After a few days your body will become used to the amount and will start to ask for more by making you thirsty. You must be sure to spread this intake of water over the whole day – drinking it all in one go will put pressure on your internal organs and is not healthy. Reduce the amount you drink leading up to bedtime so that you won't have to get up during the night. You will eventually, after about seven days, feel how much water you require. If you are feeling bloated, then reduce the water intake a little, perhaps by 250 ml (9 fl oz) or increase it by the same amount if you are still thirsty. You will be able to determine your own personal, comfortable intake levels.

'At first it was difficult to get used to eating very different types of food and I was also surprised how long it took me to get used to no caffeine – I had a mild headache for nearly five days, which indicated just how much I used to drink without thinking about it. It was all worth it as I have never felt livelier, brighter or more energised.'

Joyce, London

Superfoods These foods are generally high in nutritional value and can act as real boosters in any detox programme as well as being part of a general healthy-eating plan. For this reason, the following list of foods must feature in your daily intake.

I am not suggesting you eat every superfood, every day, but they should feature in some way, either as an ingredient in a recipe or as a snack, as often as possible. Vary them from day to day, for interest and taste. Any of the foods below can be taken in any form: raw or cooked, as a juice or tea, in a supplement (but fresh is best), as a snack or as part of a main meal:

Garlic boosts your immune system, improves circulation, reduces cholesterol, good liver tonic, reduces high blood pressure.

Grapes Powerful antioxidant, protect the heart and are good for the circulation, high in water and fibre, good liver tonic.

Onions stabilise blood sugar levels, help reduce risk of heart disease, relieve congestions in airways, boost immunity.

Beetroot Cleansing and detoxifying, good for circulation, boosts immune system, strengthens blood by building up red blood cells, fights infection, energises and balances through its iron and natural sugar content, reduces inflammation.

Carrots lower blood cholesterol, increase levels of beta-carotene in the body, boost immune system, help to heal ulcers, good for teeth, hair and bones, improve condition of skin and reduce wrinkles, good liver tonic, promote general all-round health, good for the blood, heart and circulation, good for the eyes – and of course, we all know they 'help you see in the dark'!

Fennel aids digestion, eases intestinal cramps, regulates hormone levels, eases fluid retention and flatulence, helps regulate high blood pressure due to its high potassium levels.

Manuka (or organic) honey fights bacteria, provides natural energy, softening for the skin if applied topically, protects the immune system, soothes throat problems, coughs, colds and respiratory infections; relieves stomach upset.

Blueberries improve circulation, boost immune system, good antioxidant, anti-inflammatory.

Broccoli lowers risk of heart disease, lowers risk of cataracts, combats anaemia, high in nutrients and anti-oxidants, good for the digestive system and liver, mood enhancer, good for skin, contains high concentrations of folic acid for strengthening nervous system and blood. Broccoli is one of the all-round superfoods; get a taste for it now, raw dipped in hummus is delicious and unbelievably good for you.

Spinach Antioxidant, lowers risk of heart disease, may aid in reduction of progression of age-related macular degeneration, high in folates, good source of iron, relieves anaemia, high in potassium which regulates blood pressure. (Eat two or three times a week, not every day.)

Tomatoes   Strong antioxidant due to levels of lycopene, can help to prevent many illnesses from heart conditions to skin cancers, thin the blood, improve digestion, strengthen immunity, reduce liver inflammation, reported to reduce the risk of prostate cancer. Another good all-rounder, fabulous with a delicious salad dressing and one of the few foods that doesn't seem to lose any of its potency through cooking, tinned tomatoes being as good for you as raw.

Watercress boosts the immune system, protects against heart illness, good for teeth, skin, bones, muscles, heart and nervous system, great energy booster.

Cabbage (including red) Strong antioxidant, can reduce risk of cancers, good for the heart, improves digestion and digestive health, fights bacteria, tones liver, boosts immunity.

> 'I have so much more energy. For the first time in years I feel as if my body is firing on all cylinders.'
>
> *P. Thomas, London*

Multivitamin supplements   Vitamin supplements will ensure that any problems or shortfalls in the early stages of the programme will not leave the body short of essential nutrients. This is especially helpful if you are making substantial changes to your eating habits. But after 15 days you can stop as, by this stage, your body will be getting all essential nutrients from the programme.

Three meals a day   Eating three meals a day is

becoming less and less common: we tend to skip breakfast, have lunch on the hoof and grab supper late at night. During the programme you must eat a minimum of three meals every day but, preferably, five smaller meals.

Ideally, breakfast should be before 9 a.m., lunch before 2 p.m. and the evening meal before 7 p.m. This allows sufficient time for your body to process the food before the next meal, and to process all the foods eaten that day before the start of the following day. (In a healthy body foods should normally take less than 24 hours to go from eating to defecation, but most people take more than twice that time to process what they eat.)

Brown rice   Rice is one of the most absorbent carbohydrates we can have in our diet. It also seems not to give rise to the allergic reactions and intolerances that many wheat-based carbohydrates cause. Being absorbent, it can act as a 'plunger' for our intestines. Imagine your household pipes after 20 years of use – it is likely that they have either corroded or you have had to call in a plumber to sort out minor and major blockages. As rice travels through the gut it collects all the silt and waste on the way and then flushes it out. And when you are detoxing, it means that each time waste is removed in this way it is not replaced – each time you eat absorbent rice it will break away a little more of the accumulated waste until the gut is completely cleansed.

Short grain brown rice is the most absorbent kind and should be used throughout the programme. If there are occasions, for instance, when eating out and short grain is not available, then long grain brown or wild rice are the next best options.

Other foods on the detox list The remaining ingredients in all your meals will consist entirely of fruit, vegetables, salads, herbs, fish, nuts, beans, pulses, seeds and goat's or sheep's cheeses/yogurts and so on, or their vegan equivalent. In order to get a healthy spread of necessary nutrients you must have some of each of these foods every day. If you miss out on a food category you may begin to feel lethargic, as something essential to your daily requirements will be missing. You don't need to have everything for every meal but a sensible combination could be fruit for breakfast, nuts for a mid-morning snack, fish salad for lunch, roast vegetables and rice for supper and goat's cheese and rice cakes for dessert. Try to vary this as much as possible, but make sure you eat it all. It is important to include raw foods as well as lightly cooked foods, for raw foods provide bulk and fibre that will increase the body's ability to detox.

> 'I discovered the joy of early mornings – I woke at least an hour earlier, refreshed and ready to go!'
>
> *F. Wheatley, Devon*

THE FOOD LISTS

Fruit, vegetables and salad: the specifics

High in nutrients, fruit, vegetables and salads contain large amounts of essential vitamins, amino acids and minerals. They have a high fibre and high potassium content, but contain very little waste and very few calories. Fruit, vegetables and salads consist nearly entirely of goodness. You should aim to eat fruit, vegetables and salads as fresh as possible. The longer you store them the more nutrients are lost, and, certainly, as soon as you begin to process them yourself the goodness will disappear quickly. Raw food equates to raw energy; raw food cleans the gut more efficiently; and raw food contains high levels of dietary fibre. So you should attempt to eat as much of your fruit and vegetable quota in its raw state. If this is impossible then make sure that a high percentage is raw. For instance, salad with lightly steamed vegetables, or grated raw carrot and beetroot over a bowl of grilled vegetables. Fruit can be eaten fresh or dried. Try juicing your vegetables for one of your daily portions.

The fruit list

All berries, including bilberries, blackberries, blueberries, cranberries, gooseberries, loganberries, raspberries, strawberries

Apples

Apricots

Bananas

Blackcurrants

Cherries

Currants (dried and fresh)

Damsons

Dates

Figs

Grapefruit

Grapes

Greengages

Guavas

Kiwi fruit

Lemons

Limes

Lychees

Mangoes

Melons

Mulberries

Nectarines

Passion fruit

Paw-paw

Peaches

Pears

Pineapple

Plums

Pomegranates

Prunes

Quinces

Raisins

Redcurrants

Rhubarb

Sultanas

The vegetable list

Artichokes, globe
and Jerusalem
Asparagus
Aubergines (eggplant)
Beans, French,
runner, broad,
butter, haricot
Bean sprouts
Beetroot
Broccoli
Brussels sprouts
Cabbage, red, Savoy
Carrots
Cauliflower
Celeriac
Celery

Chicory
Chinese leaf
Courgettes (zucchini)
Cucumber
Fennel
Kohlrabi
Leeks
Lettuce, all types
Marrow
Okra (ladies' fingers)
Onions
Parsnips
Peas, all types
Peppers (bell peppers,
capsicums)
Plantain

Potatoes
Pumpkin
Radishes
Spring greens
Spring onions
(scallions)
Squash, spring, white
and winter
Swede
Sweetcorn (corn on
the cob, maize)
Sweet potatoes
Tomatoes
Turnips
Watercress
Yams

Nuts: the specifics

Although high in calories, nuts are also extremely high in
nutrients, an excellent source of essential unsaturated
fatty acids and are a rich source of potassium and fibre.
You can eat any nuts, but here is a short list. They should
be eaten raw, unsalted and fresh.

The nut list

Almonds
Brazil nuts
Cashew nuts
Chestnuts

Hazelnuts
Macadamia nuts
Pecan nuts
Pine nuts

Pistachio nuts
Walnuts

Beans, grains, pulses, seeds, herbs and spices: the specifics

Beans and pulses are full of nutrients – in fact – full of beans. If they are dried, they can be soaked overnight, but, for convenience, you can use tinned versions as long as you rinse off the brine or juice they come in.

Sprouted beans and seeds are high in nutrients and once they are freshly sprouted the nutrient content becomes even higher. When a seed has sprouted it is easier to digest, as the process of sprouting starts to break it down, which means there is less work for our digestive system to do. Seeds and sprouts add flavour and colour to our foods, but their vitamin and nutrient content is of ultimate importance.

Herbs should ideally be fresh so that you get the benefit of all their nutrients. Dried herbs will supply flavour but little else. Grains and spices add flavour and texture and the hotter spices can be very stimulating for the digestion. The total list is very long, but a few are included in the list below.

The beans, grains, pulse, seed, herb and spice list

Aduki	Dill	Pumpkin seeds
Alfalfa	Fennel	Quinoa, white and red
Basil	Ginger, fresh	Rosemary
Black beans	and powdered	Sage
Cardamom pods	Kidney	Sesame seeds
Cayenne pepper	Lemon grass	Soy/edamane, ground
Chick peas	Lentils, puy, normal	Split peas
Chillies	Marjoram	Sunflower seeds
Coriander, fresh	Parsley	Tarragon
and powdered	Pepper, fresh	Thyme

Non-dairy: the specifics

The odd term, non-dairy, best describes the fermentation process, which is different from that used in cow's milk production. The process means that goat's and sheep's products are much easier to digest and can also aid digestive disorders and actually stimulate digestion. Many people who have developed an allergy or intolerance to cow's milk products will not necessarily have a reaction to either sheep's or goat's milk products.

The non-dairy list

Goat's cheese	Sheep's milk	Rice milk
Sheep's cheese	Goat's yogurt	Soya milk
Goat's milk	Sheep's yogurt	

Fish: the specifics

All fish contain essential proteins, but oily fish such as herrings, mackerel and salmon has the added benefit of the omega 3 fatty acids. Wherever possible you should eat fresh fish. If fresh is not available or you are using canned fish for convenience, the best varieties are those canned in olive or vegetable oil. Some fish is canned in spring water, so check that no salt has been added. If it has, then make sure the fish is drained completely and rinsed before eating. Fish in brine is the same, drain as much as possible before eating. Smoked fish is acceptable but should be naturally smoked and not dyed or coloured. Frozen can be used for convenience, but breadcrumbs are a push too far! Fresh is always best and will contain the most nutrients. You can eat any fish, but here are some readily available types.

The fish list

Cod	Mackerel	Scampi
Crab	Monkfish	Shrimps
Haddock	Pilchards	Skate
Halibut	Plaice	Trout
Herring	Prawns	Tuna
Lemon sole	Salmon	
Lobster	Sardines	

Drinks: the specifics

During the programme you are required to drink 1.5 litres (2¾ pints) of water per day. If the water becomes a little repetitive you can use some natural flavourings to make it more interesting. Try honey or lemon. Juices are not counted as water but can be drunk in addition to the required amounts. If you are buying ready-squeezed juices, try to get pure juice in preference to juice made up in water from fruit pulp – it will say on the carton or bottle. If you are drinking juices, they are very concentrated so always dilute 50/50 with water.

The drinks list

Herbal teas, any	Juices freshly squeezed,	Water, hot, cold,
Honey in water	pure and	fizzy and spring,
Lemon juice in	unsweetened,	with tap water
water	apple or grape or	for emergencies
	any juiced vegetable	only

Miscellaneous foods: the specifics

These are the items that are hard to categorise. They are, however, just as essential to the programme as the foods listed earlier, as, they too, add nutrients, variety and flavour. Try to include as many of these as possible. Tahini can be bought from most health food stores. You can choose between 'light' tahini, sesame seeds that are hulled before being ground, or 'dark' tahini, which simply means that the hulls have been left on. Make sure that your tahini is unsalted – most are, but it is worth checking on the ingredients.

It is worth pointing out at this stage that you should get yourself down to your local health food store and start to read labels. As long as there is nothing added, such as sugars and salts, there are lots of natural foods that are easy to use and will enhance your detox programme: mushroom pâtés, tinned bean sprouts, chestnut purées. These are foods that you would not automatically think of and are far too numerous to list here, but they are perfectly suitable for the programme.

The miscellaneous list

Balsamic vinegar
Cider vinegar
Grapeseed oil
Guacamole
Miso soup, paste
Mustard, grain,
 not powder

Oats
Olive oil
Olives, green
 or black
Pumpkin seed oil
Quorn
Raspberry balsamic
 vinegar

Rice cakes, unsalted
Seaweed
Sesame oil
Tahini
Tofu
Walnut oil

Common foods you cannot have in the first week

There are many foods that are very good for you, but for the detox programme, and as we tend to eat a lot of them, they are excluded in the early stages, mainly because they could tip the balance while we are changing our eating habits and may interfere with the intestinal balance in the early stages of your programme. You can introduce them after the first week and munch away to your heart's content!

For example; oranges are on the list because they are the most acidic of all fruit. But, their close relatives, however (tangerines, satsumas and so on), are less acidic and can be included on the Detox Programme throughout. Acidity is harmful to the liver, and foods containing large amounts of acids should be avoided. Contrary to what you might think, grapefruit, limes and lemons are all alkaline-producing foods and so are included throughout the programme.

Foods not to be eaten in the first week

While these foods are excluded in the first week because of the reasons listed below, they are acceptable in moderation after Day 7.

Avocados	*High in starch and fat and we tend to eat loads if we like them*
Bananas	*High in starch and fat and we tend to eat too many if we like them*
Lentils	*Can produce too much gas. If you do find when you introduce them, that you are a little bit windy, then really limit your intake, or eat brown short grain rice instead for your bulk. It's*

	the same with pulses, if they have this effect, then restrict consumption.
Mushrooms	*Too much fungus*
Oranges	*High acidity*
Peanuts	*High in fat and starch*

Banned foods

There are some foods and drinks that are most definitely banned from your diet during your detox programme. They have a negative nutritional value, are hard to digest, or are found naturally in other foods so we do not have to add more. The list isn't that long, but they are foods we perhaps eat too much of.

Alcohol	*It's good to spend a month without!*
Bread, pasta, refined white rice	*Gluten in the wheat flour can be difficult to digest, and some people are intolerant (their bodies have difficulty digesting it easily).*
Caffeine	*Chemical stimulant.*
Chocolate	*Too much sugar and fat.*
Cow's milk/cheese etc.	*Lactose (milk sugar) can be difficult to digest.*
Added salt	*Naturally found in foods, and too much salt results in potassium deficiency and water retention.*
Added sugar	*Naturally found in foods, too much sugar disturbs blood glucose levels, causing disturbed appetite and energy levels, naturally found in foods.*
Colourings/preservatives, and E numbers	*No nutritional value.*
Red and white meat	*Fish is the healthiest animal protein for this programme.*
Fizzy drinks/cordials etc.	*No nutritional value.*

As you can see, the choice of available foods on the Detox Programme is extensive, so there is absolutely no excuse to stray from it. If you choose to use only a small selection of the foods available you will still be able to follow an interesting and varied programme, and those that you do not eat you can save for next time.

ADDITIONAL INFORMATION ON FOOD

Portion sizes

The Detox Programme is very specifically named – it is a programme and not a diet. A portion is a heaped tablespoon. A portion of fish is a fillet or steak, a portion of seafood a tablespoon and a portion of cheese is two to three ounces (50–75g).

Each meal will include a combination of at least three portions of either rice, vegetables or miscellaneous foods. Each meal should be a full plate or bowl. If at any stage you get hungry you must eat something, even if this means you are eating more than your three to five small meals per day, especially in the first half of the programme as your body adjusts. You are likely to think you are eating more than you should, but this is normal and correct.

Balanced diet

Vegetables, salads, fruit and rice provide a great source of carbohydrates and fibre, while fish, oil and nuts are good sources of protein and fats. You must make sure that at least two portions of foods such as olive oil, cashew nuts and oily fish are included every day or your programme will lack the necessary balance – you are not eating any of your normal fats, so adding (beneficial) oils is crucial. If you just eat vegetables, salads, rice and fruit you will get tired and your detox process will slow down to a stop.

Calorie intake

The Detox Programme is not calorie-counted, but calories are a good way of demonstrating how much you need to eat. Calories are a measure of the amount of energy in our food. The average woman should eat around 1,600 calories per day and men 2000, and never go below 1,000 calories, even when dieting. If the calorie intake is reduced below 1,000 per day we are not providing sufficient energy for our bodies to operate properly and we go into starvation mode. Although our bodies store fat for times, such as this, when it is needed, our metabolism slows down and we become weak and lethargic. It is imperative that during the programme you don't let your intake go below the recommended calorie intake per day: the detox will only work if you keep all your organs and systems functioning healthily.

Cooking techniques

While on the Detox Programme you should try to cook your foods as little as possible. The less heat the food is subjected to, the more nutrients will remain. Obviously all fish dishes need to be cooked thoroughly, but cooked vegetables should always be eaten slightly crisp and al dente. Techniques such as light steaming, parboiling, microwaving, stir-frying or flash-frying and grilling are much preferable to boiling, deep-fat frying or slow cooking, which destroy both flavour and nutrients.

Using your imagination

You have an extensive list of individual fresh foods, and what you need to do now is to start using your imagination. Just because the list contains lots of individual items doesn't mean that you cannot combine them to make many commonly used foods – without any processing, additives, preservatives, and so on. Here are some basic examples of what you can include if you use foods from the lists and a little imagination.

Hummus

Garlic, olive oil, sesame seed paste (tahini), lemon juice and chick peas are all on the list. In Chapter 5 you will find a recipe for turning these ingredients into the most delicious home-made hummus you have ever tasted. Hummus is good for late-night snacks and for satisfying emergency hunger pangs.

Salad dressings

Olive oil, sesame oil, cider vinegar, lime juice, wholegrain mustard and pepper are all on the list. Chapter 5 will offer you a refreshingly sharp dressing for your salads. There are also many shops now that sell the most exotic natural oils and dressings; my current favourites are walnut oil with raspberry vinegar or pumpkin seed oil, also with same raspberry vinegar. A small amount of dressing goes a long way and it totally transforms a simple salad in seconds. This is the time to get your taste buds working and discover some fabulous new eating habits and taste sensations.

Entertaining

Having friends for supper is easy on the Detox Programme. Fish, olives, herbs and vegetables are all on the list, and a meal of grilled fish with a herb and olive crust on a bed of chargrilled vegetables drizzled with walnut oil is a gastronomic treat at any time. There are so many other combinations among the recipes in Chapter 5 that your guests would find it hard to believe if you told them they were 'detoxing'.

Top secret!

Now, I am human, I have done this programme many, many times. I do it in February as there are 28 days and I also have two major occasions in this month, my partner's birthday and St Valentine's day. I am realistic, and if I told you I had *never* cheated on the programme, I wouldn't be being totally honest with you. I use the word 'cheated' wisely, because I know it's me I am cheating; but then the human mind is fabulous in that I can consider my mind able to cheat my body – like the two aren't both part of me!

So, for this reason, I am going to share with you the 'falling off the wagon/illegal foods list'. Over your 30-day programme you can have the following as an emergency measure. Please do not exceed the total amount on the list during the programme, it is not an everyday allowance.

Emergency measures (for the whole 30 days, so if you have had them all by Day 5, that's it).

- 1 50g bar of chocolate – at least 60 per cent cocoa content.

- 2 small glasses of wine.

- 2 pieces of toast, wholegrain or wholemeal please.

- 2 portions of white meat, chicken or turkey, not pork.

- 2 portions white rice.

- 2 small bags of vegetable crisps (parsnips/carrots/mixed veg).

This should help you get through those moments that you find totally unavoidable – and there's not much on the list, so don't think I'm letting you off, it just helps in moments of madness for you not to think you have ruined your programme. For those chocaholics, I would rather you had one small square of high-quality cocoa every now and then than a candy bar or cake hidden behind the filing cabinets.

If savoury is your thing, then vegetable crisps should see you through – they are not on the programme because of the added salt, and so on. This small concession to your cravings should keep the snack attack for a whole bag of tortillas at bay.

So that's it, our secret stash of survival foods ... shhh!

On to the Next Stage

Now that you have the food basics we need to look at the body-care basics and recipe suggestions. In later chapters we shall look at all the ways to enhance the programme further and to pamper yourself during it.

It is very important to carry out the body-care section of the programme, as it is designed to enhance and speed up the detox process. The treatments enhance the programme because they complement everything that you will be doing for yourself during the next 30 days. Don't think they are a luxury just because they are nice – make sure you realise they are a necessity.

> 'My hair and fingernails have grown like wildfire, I've lost a lot of excess fluid so my legs feel lighter, my stomach is flat as a board. I feel squeaky-clean and vital.'
>
> *Kate, London*

Body Care and the Detox Programme

The Detox Programme is all you will ever need to keep your body in the best possible condition from within. The nutrients from the foods, the internal cleansing actions of the rice, lemon water, fluids and so on, the cleansing of the eliminatory organs, the supplements, superfoods and 'everyday foods' will all provide a fully rounded internal cleanse. The Detox Programme is also the main and most important way to keep your body in the best possible condition from the outside. But there is much more to do to enhance the vitality of your body and mind through a daily and weekly body-care routine.

During the Detox Programme, from Day 1 to Day 30 you must:

- Do dry-skin brushing every morning.

- Take a cool shower every morning.

- Self-massage every morning and evening.

- Take 20 minutes' exercise every day.

- Have ten minutes' relaxation every day.

- Have five minutes of quality breathing every day.

- Say five affirmations or do five visualisations ten times each day.

- Smile or laugh heartily every day.

- Exfoliate every three days.

- Take a mineral-salt bath every five days.

> 'What I hadn't expected was that my skin would feel so soft – it glowed with health after only three weeks.'
> *S. Payne, London*

THE DAILY TREATMENTS

Cool showers

Now, I used to be very mean about instructing on how to take a cool shower, I just told everyone to turn the water to cold and stand there! No wonder some people found it a challenge too far. Well, I am much better educated now on hydrotherapy – hot and cold showers to you and me – and the instructions below should make the whole experience not only a lot more acceptable but also much more effective.

An invigorating swim in a cool pool, sea or lake every morning would be an ideal scenario. The cold water will increase your circulation, tone your muscles and skin and give the lymph a jump-start. But if you needed to include a long, cool swim every day on the Detox Programme, alongside all your other new activities, you would soon find that you would be spending more time detoxing and less time living your life! The alternative takes two minutes and has all the benefits of the swim without having to leave your own home – just take a cool shower.

This may sound mad, but if you have ever taken a shower or bath in a place where there was no hot water you will remember that it was a most invigorating experience that actually left you considerably warmer than it would if you had taken a normal hot shower. Indeed, in hot weather it is more effective to take a shower that is lukewarm or at blood temperature rather than a cold shower; the latter will increase your circulation and warm you up rather than cool you down.

The healing powers of cool showers are phenomenal:

they boost your circulation, boost your immune system, tone your muscles and tone your skin. They are very good at temperature regulation for your body, so if any of you are nearing that certain age when hot flushes are becoming part of your day, then the following instructions should be followed, without doubt, every day. Whatever your situation, you will very soon notice an amazing difference.

Try any of the following routines and see which one suits you best. Remember you are required to take some kind of temperature bathing every day – so mix and match or find your favourite.

Any of these treatments can be done twice a day, but not at the same time. You can do one in the morning and one in the evening if you like.

Not everyone reacts to temperature the same way. The degrees of hot and cold will vary greatly, but they must feel hot to you and cool to you for it to work.

It is up to you to determine how hot and how cold something needs to be in order for your body to respond to the extreme temperatures in a positive yet challenging way.

Alternating shower

Good for the heart and all-over relief of pain, rejuvenation and lymph detox. This is a powerful treatment, not to be underestimated and it doesn't cost much! (If you do not have a shower head that you can detach from the wall and adjust, then use a water jug or bowl for the cold application of this treatment.)

1. Take a hot shower, stay in the hot shower until you feel nice and warm.

2. Step out of the flow of the water.

3. Turn the shower to cold and keep holding the flow of water away from your body.

4. In the following order pour cold water over your body.

5. On your right leg pour cold water from ankle to the hip on the outside of the leg.

6. On your right leg pour cold water from ankle to hip on the inside of the leg.

7. Repeat this on your left leg.

If this was a real challenge, then just do this bit for five days. By then you will be ready to add your arms for the next five days.

1. On your right arm pour cold water from wrist to the shoulder on the outside of the arm.

2. On your right arm pour cold water from wrist to shoulder on the inside of the arm.

3. Repeat this on your left arm.

If this was a challenge, then do legs and arms for the next five days and then introduce your body for the next five days.

1. Pour cold water up the front of your body from hips to neck.

2. Pour cold water down your back from neck to hips.

If this was a challenge then stay with legs, arms and body for the next five days and then introduce your head – and so do your whole body – for the final days of the programme.

• Pour cold water over your face and head.

You may do the sequence just once each day, but to make it much more effective, repeat the process three times, finishing with the cool water.

Whatever stage you are at, when you have completed the procedure, step out of the shower and dry off. If you did this correctly you will be feeling quite warm and invigorated.

WATER TREADING

If cool showers are beyond you or if you do not have access to a shower, then you can do the following, using buckets or in your bath. This exercise is good for the lymphatic system and pain in the feet and legs.

1. In the bath or in the buckets, put ice-cold water deep enough to cover your lower legs

2. Stand in this ice-cold water.

3. Begin to Stork Walk (walking on the spot and bringing your knees up to your chest with each step) for a period of 1–5 minutes.

4. Step out of the ice-cold water.

5. Dry only between your toes; do not dry the feet or legs.

6. Let the feet and legs air-dry before putting on your socks and shoes.

ARM PLUNGE

If there are times when you are working at the computer, or doing physical work with your arms but you do not have access to a shower or bath, the 'arm plunge' is an effective treatment. It is good for the heart and for pain in the arms and hands.

1. In a sink or bucket put ice-cold water deep enough to cover your arms up to 10 cm (4in) over your elbows – not all the way up to your shoulders.

2. Your arms should be bent as if you are resting in the sink or bucket of ice-cold water.

3. Hold your arms in this water for 1–3 minutes – no more.

4. Bring your arms out of the ice-cold water and brush off the excess water.

5. Do not dry your arms, let them air-dry.

Dry-skin brushing

This once-unheard-of process now bounces from every health article you read – and quite right too! Sloughing away dead skin cells helps remove any barriers to your skin 'breathing' efficiently. It clears the pores and improves the appearance of the skin – dead skin is dull and does not reflect light well, whereas healthy skin glows in normal light conditions. Brushing also stimulates the production of sebum, which, in turn, helps to improve the texture and tone of the skin.

Brushing improves blood and lymph circulation by stimulating muscle contraction. The improved lymph flow causes more efficient excretion of waste materials in the cells and interstitial fluids occurring in the spaces between organs and tissues. Clearing this area encourages more efficient cell production and renewal. Increasing the flow of interstitial fluid also causes excess fluids to drain and clear from the more troublesome areas of the hips and thighs. Pooling of fluid around the ankles, lower back or lower neck, water retention or oedema can be prevented with more efficient fluid and lymph flow.

Effective brushing

Now that you have plenty of excellent reasons to dry-skin brush, the next step is to know how to do it effectively.

1. Take a natural-bristle brush, a loofah, a dry flannel or mitt. Whichever you use should be firm but not hard, as you will be brushing your skin quite vigorously all over your body. The skin on your stomach, for instance, is softer than the skin on your shins or fore-arms. Do not wet or moisturise the skin, as this may cause dragging.

2. Undress to your underwear or, preferably, take all your clothes off. Stand or sit in a position that gives you access to all parts of your body – the edge of the bed with your feet up on pillows is quite good, or you can sit on the edge of the bath with one foot up on the toilet seat if it is close enough.

3. Start at your feet and systematically work up towards the top of your body. All strokes should be towards the heart – the heart is a wonderful machine for pumping the blood down and out to all parts of the body, but both blood and lymph need extra help to work against gravity to return through the system. If you brush away from the heart it may cause faintness or disrupt the normal flow. Each stroke should be long and firm. Place the brush/mitt on your ankle and firmly brush up to your knee, then repeat until you have covered the entire calf and shin several times. When you have completed the lower leg, move up to the knee. The next set of strokes should run from the knee to the top of the thigh and over the buttocks.

4. Then brush both arms, from the wrist to the shoulder. The neck and shoulder area should be treated more gently as the flesh here is very delicate. Work from the top of your arm, up and over your shoulder and gently up your neck to the base of your skull.

5. When brushing your stomach, use gentle circular strokes in a clockwise direction. This will follow the flow in your intestines and will not disrupt any bowel functions.

6. You must only brush your face with a soft facial brush or flannel, as the skin here is very delicate and can be damaged if the brush is too hard.

The whole process should take only three or four minutes and afterwards you should feel invigorated. Your skin will tingle and you should feel quite warm as you will have stimulated and increased your circulation. After only a few sessions you will notice quite a difference in your skin – it feels smoother, with a softer texture, and the dry patches will have all disappeared. Just spend a little time each day and you will be pleasantly surprised.

Self-massage

I could go on for days about how good massage is for everything! There is a full description of the methods and benefits on pages 214–217, so I will limit what I say here to the more specific ways that massage can enhance the detox process. Everything we know about the benefits of massage is true for self-massage. It would be wonderful if we could all have massage treatments every day of our lives, but it takes time and money. Self-massage avoids all these problems: it is cheap and can be done any time or anywhere. Since daily massage is required on the 30-day programme, self-massage is essential.

So why is massage so good for detox? This list is just for starters – there are many more beneficial effects:

- It warms and relaxes our muscles.

- It relieves tension.

- It helps to reduce stress.

- It increases blood circulation.

- It increases lymph flow.

- It helps to improve the immune system.

- It helps the body to eliminate excess fluids.

- It helps the body to eliminate waste products.

- It improves the flow of interstitial fluid, improving the appearance of the skin, especially in areas that are prone to cellulite.

- It lowers blood pressure.

- It tones the muscles.

- It tones the skin.

- It is a passive workout for the whole body.

Self-massage techniques

Most normal massage strokes can be converted for self-massage. As long as you observe the general rules of massage, even 'made-up' strokes will be perfectly accept-able and effective.

- As with dry-skin brushing, all massage strokes should be towards the heart, pushing the blood around the system in conjunction with the circulation and not against it.

- All strokes should be using either the flat hand (fingers together, palms down) or with the ends of the fingers (bunched together, no fingernails).

- All massage strokes should start lightly and slowly build to a firmer, more rapid pace.

- Your flesh should be warm and relaxed before any

deeper strokes can be used. Working deeply on cold, tense flesh will feel unpleasant and cause bruising.

- Massage should never be painful or sore, but massage that is too light is little better than a comforting stroke.

- You should be relaxed when carrying out self-massage, as you need to work in some awkward positions and do not want to cause any twists or injuries.

You should massage yourself every day during the Detox Programme, but as this can become time-consuming I have broken down the massage sequence into smaller elements. Try to do at least two of the elements every day to ensure that over each week you will get a full-body treatment. Remember, take it slowly at first. Then, as your knowledge and confidence build, you will be able to make adjustments as necessary.

Where possible you should make sure that the room you are in is warm and quiet, perhaps with some relaxing or calming music. If the room is cold it is likely that you will not be totally relaxed, which will not result in the best massage.

You should use a massage oil, favourite cream or body lotion and apply just enough to allow your hands to work over the flesh firmly. If you use too much you will just slip over the skin, and if you use too little you may pull or 'burn' the skin. Reapply as necessary. If you apply too much, just wipe the excess on another part of your body until you need it later.

Face and neck sequence

Place the pads of your fingers together and press them onto your face quite firmly. Working together, circle both hands upwards, out and down, all over the surface of your face – remember to work the cheeks, forehead, nose, lips and so on. Then relax your jawbone and let your mouth relax. Continue strokes down your neck and over the front of your chest in small and large circles.

Shoulder and arm sequence

Place your hand flat onto your lower arm. Keeping as much of your hand as possible on the arm, work in long, smooth, firm strokes from the base of the arm, up and over the shoulder. The pressure should be on the upward stroke, and released on the downward stroke. What you are doing is pushing the blood up towards the top of your arm.

Hand and wrist sequence

Place the thumb of your left hand on the knuckle of your right thumb. 'Drain' the blood and lymph from your knuckle to your wrist in long, smooth strokes. Repeat with all knuckles on that hand until you have 'drained' the entire hand and wrist. Firm pressure is required from the start to the end of each stroke. Do the same for your left hand.

Stomach and chest sequence

Place your hands flat on your stomach and massage both of them in large circles over the entire torso. The right hand should travel anticlockwise and the left hand clockwise, with firm strokes.

Lower back and spine sequence

Stand with your legs shoulder-width apart. Place your hands on your hips with the fingers in front and the thumbs on your back. Press your thumbs firmly into your spine and lower back and move in deep, firm circles. Cover as much of the spine area as possible.

Thigh and buttock sequence

Sit with your legs supported on the side of the bed or bath or with pillows underneath them. Working on one leg at a time, use flat hands to work in firm circles over the entire buttock and thigh area. Once the flesh becomes warm and slightly pink, clench your fist and continue with the firm circles. Work gently at first and build the pressure slowly.

Calf and foot sequence

Placing both hands flat on the tops of your feet, brush them up towards your knees in long, firm strokes. Repeat rapidly several times. Move your hands to the back of your leg and press the flesh firmly, lifting it and pushing it alternately. Work the flesh backwards and forwards, taking care not to 'burn' it.

EXERCISE

This is one of the best ways to enhance the Detox Programme. It costs nothing, it can be done at any time of the day or night, even while you are doing everyday chores, and it can have many, many benefits. As far back as the early 90s, the 'then' Fitness Association in the UK (now the Fitness Industry Association) issued a list of reasons why exercise is good for you, and the ones in italics are particularly relevant to the Detox Programme. The information has not changed in relevance; exercise is STILL good for you!

- Promotes increased stamina
- Relieves symptoms of menopause
- May help prevent heart disease
- Prevents osteoporosis
- Reduces the risk of breast cancer
- Lessens arthritis pain
- Controls cholesterol
- Burns fat
- *Speeds up metabolism*
- Alleviates PMT
- Helps you to stop smoking
- Relieves depression
- Releases anxiety
- Improves sexual performance
- Improves mental sharpness
- Improves concentration
- Improves outlook
- Reduces medical costs
- Increases job satisfaction
- Preserves muscle
- Preserves internal organs (liver, kidneys)
- Improves reaction time
- Increases range of motion
- *Improves cardiovascular fitness*
- *Increases energy*
- Improves neuromuscular (nerve and muscle) coordination
- Increases the body's ability to fight off infection.
- Reduces the risk of glaucoma
- Decreases the risk of colon cancer
- Lowers blood pressure
- Reduces the risk of obesity
- Burns calories
- *Relieves constipation*
- Prevents endometriosis
- Reduces alcohol consumption
- Reduces stress
- *Enhances self-esteem*
- *Heightens sense of wellbeing*
- Increases IQ
- Enhances creativity
- Decreases job absenteeism
- Increases productivity
- Improves flexibility
- *Improves circulation*
- Increases mobility
- Improves memory
- Shortens recovery time after illness or injury
- Promotes a healthy back
- *Deepens sleep*
- *Lengthens life*

You should do at least 20 minutes' exercise every day during your detox programme. Not only will this help to keep you fit and toned, but it will also ensure that your metabolic rate does not decrease or your circulation become sluggish.

A little and often is much better than spending two hours every two weeks. The latter is likely to tire you out more quickly; also, you will not build up any benefit from your exercise as it happens too infrequently, which in turn will be discouraging and you may well give up. If you exercise for 20 minutes every day it doesn't interfere with your day too much, it's over before you get bored and you will notice the benefits after just a few days. So you are much more likely to get inspired and start extending to 30 and then 40 minutes, until you build up to a level of exercise that naturally suits you and your lifestyle.

Getting started is the hardest part. Think about how your day works and how you can slip in the exercise without even noticing:

- If you normally start by going downstairs to get the post or to make breakfast, go up and down the stairs three times before you actually boil the kettle.

- If you normally drive to pick up the children from school, then walk (it will do the children good, too).

- As you are cleaning the house you could jog while vacuuming or stretch for five minutes while dusting.

- If you are going to be sitting in a meeting for several hours, go to the meeting room via the longest route and run up the stairs several times before sitting down.

- In the evening while watching the television you can lift and lower your legs, or tense and relax your stomach muscles several times.

- When everyone is out of the house, put on some music and dance for 20 minutes – this feels great and is excellent exercise as well.

- Don't go out to the pub – go to a nightclub and dance.

- Go rollerblading rather than walking on Sunday.

- Don't watch the kids in the pool – get in there with them.

- Sit in the bath and do stretches from side to side or scissor your legs together and apart using the water as weights – but be careful not to splash too much!

Of course, the more traditional methods of exercise are still very valuable – joining a gymnasium, going to exercise classes, playing sport, jogging, and so on. But if you have tried all these and not found an exercise you're happy with, don't be discouraged. Set yourself a challenge to find the most unusual form of exercise you can, and do it for 30 minutes each day.

If you are the type of person who likes to follow sequences, get a video exercise tape of someone whom you like and admire and work with this, gradually building up the amount of time you spend until you can do the whole tape without blinking. Also, the following pages will take you through an elementary routine that you can do yourself.

Exercise sequence

1. Walk up and down ten steps or stairs for five minutes at a normal pace.

2. Stand with feet shoulder-width apart and alternately lift your left leg and left arm up and out to the side, then your right leg and right arm up and out to the side. Repeat ten times each side. NB: Keep your arms and knees slightly bent.

3. Standing in the same position as before, clasp your hands in front of your nose with your arms slightly bent. Keeping your shoulders relaxed, twist slowly from side to side. The stretch will gradually increase and you should end it when you can see directly behind yourself. Feel the stretch in your stomach and waist muscles. Repeat ten times each side.

4. Walk on the spot for five minutes, making sure that you bring each knee up to hip level. Swing your arms up and down in a marching style, bringing your hands up to shoulder height.

5. Walk on the spot for five minutes, bringing your knees up and out to the side to hip level. Clasp your hands in front of you with your forearms and elbows together, and as you step lift your arms and lower them. Don't let your arms drop below shoulder height.

6. Jog on the spot for five minutes without lifting your toes from the floor. You should be just lifting your heels up and down and wiggling your hips as much as possible.

7. Facing forward, twist your head slowly from side to side, looking over your right and left shoulders alternately. Hold the stretch for a moment, then release and look over the other shoulder.

8. Standing with feet shoulder-width apart, hold the back of an upright chair and lower your body until your knees are bent at 90 degrees. Hold this position for a count of five, then lift yourself slowly. Repeat 15 times. Remember to clench your buttocks and thighs as you lift and lower your body.

9. Kneel on the floor with your hands shoulder-width apart and flat on the floor. Walk your hands forward so that you are supporting your body weight on your hands and using your knees as a balance. Keeping your back straight, bend and lower your arms until your nose touches the floor, and then lift. Repeat ten times, slowly.

All these exercises, except the jogging, should be slow and deliberate. You should use your body weight as resistance to increase the effectiveness of the exercises. You can increase the number of repetitions as soon as you become comfortable with the programme – do them for as long as you wish, but for at least 30 minutes every day.

Whatever form of exercise you choose, you should treat it as something that you deserve and that enhances the Detox Programme. It is easy to think that exercise is hard work and a chore – something that both your mind and body have to endure – when actually both your body and mind love and need exercise in order to function efficiently.

Posture

Exercise is closely related to posture. We are all designed so that our internal organs have sufficient space to operate efficiently. If we change this spacing by putting on weight, losing weight, sitting with our bodies squashed or slumping while we eat, our organs need to compensate. This will lead to conditions such as: inefficient expansion of the lungs while breathing; lack of oxygen in the body; incorrect absorption of vital vitamins, minerals and food-stuffs; indigestion; poor circulation; and headaches. More obvious physical effects occur as well: slouching shoulders, weak stomach muscles and a caved-in chest. Exercise will keep the body and its muscles in good condition to prevent any of these effects occurring, or will correct any that have already set in.

Breathing

Everyone knows how important oxygen, fresh air and good breathing techniques are for us. But if you ask anyone exactly how to breathe correctly or what effects good breathing have they will probably struggle for an explanation.

Breathing correctly is fundamental to survival, and even a momentary lack of the correct level of oxygen in the body can result in serious damage and eventually death. Yet many of us continue to underuse the full capac-ity of our lungs and short-change our bodies of all the benefits that correct breathing will bring.

From early childhood we are told to 'stand up straight, stomachs in', and when we are told to take a deep breath we automatically inhale and raise our chests. But restricting movement of the stomach and abdomen means that we are limiting the area into which the lungs can expand, and so we develop the habit of using only a third of our lung capacity each time we inhale.

Balance of mind and body is also affected by breathing. If you are tense and stressed and your breathing is short and shallow you are less likely to be able to think straight, your movements become erratic and your balance is thrown.

Correct breathing is easy and more relaxing. Breathing exercises are simple and can be carried out whenever you feel it necessary.

To breathe correctly you simply relax your stomach muscles, inhale slowly through your nose and take in the air until it feels as if the base of your stomach is full of air. Then pause momentarily before exhaling through your mouth. Feeling the air 'in your stomach' shows that you have relaxed your diaphragm muscle, which means your lungs have fully expanded and you have inhaled to full capacity. This will feel strange at first, but it will soon become the normal way to breathe and you won't think about it any more.

Deeper breathing slows the heart rate and the pulse. Also, the deeper we breathe the more oxygen we inhale. All these are indications of improved and stronger health.

A simple breathing exercise

This is a good exercise to do when you feel stressed, if you cannot sleep or if you simply want to recharge your batteries.

1. Sit comfortably or lie down, supporting your lower back if necessary.

2. Place your hands on your stomach area with the fingertips just touching.

3. Start to breathe in through your nose very slowly to a count of four. As you inhale you should feel your stomach expand and your fingertips separate.

4. Hold your breath for four seconds and exhale slowly through your mouth to a count of eight.

5. Repeat several times as required.

It will feel strange at first, as you are not accustomed to using your muscles to expand your stomach in this way. However, over a period of just a few minutes it will become more natural.

Continue this exercise for at least ten inward breaths and you should feel much more relaxed and 'centred'. Eventually you will not need to use your fingers to check that your stomach is expanding rather than your chest, and soon you will be able to carry out the exercise while going about your normal day-to-day business – not the lying down, but the controlled breathing! If you ever have difficulty in dropping off to sleep this is a far more effective way than the traditional 'counting sheep'. The chances are that you won't make it to ten and will probably be asleep by six.

AFFIRMATIONS AND VISUALISATIONS

Here is a brilliant way of feeling good about yourself immediately, with long-term benefits as well. Feeling down in the dumps can be transformed into feeling positive and proactive in just a matter of moments. Once you have got into the habit of affirmations and visualisations, feeling depressed will become a thing of the past.

During the detox you can affirm your ability to complete the programme and you can visualise just how 'clean' you will be when you have finished. When you have completed the detox, when you are thinking about beginning – or just about any other time in your life – you can use affirmations and visualisations to help you.

You often hear people say, 'And if someone tells you this often enough, you really start to believe them.' That's all that affirmations are – telling yourself something, anything, often enough that you really believe it – and if you believe something it becomes real.

Affirmations don't have to be grand or extraordinary, they just have to help you. To start making affirmations you need to think about what your goal is, what you want to happen or what you want to do. It can be on any level: personal, job, home, relationship, money – anything. It is probably better to start with something small – giving up your job and living on a tropical island might be a little too adventurous for starters! And anyway, if you change something small it always leads to something bigger.

Affirmations must be positive and should be kept short. The sort of things you may want to affirm during the detox would be:

- I have a healthy body.

- I am happy with my body.

- I am cleaning my body.

- This is my month, I will enjoy looking after myself.

- I deserve to indulge myself this month.

- I am feeling great.

- I am feeling energetic.

- I am succeeding with my own personal detox.

You get the idea. Now all you have to do is repeat these to yourself or out loud. You should say them whenever they come into your mind; you can say all of them or you can say just one of them. As you are saying your affirmations you should give them positive energy, feel good about saying them and smile. You should believe that they are real and that they have come true or are coming true for you. If there is a time when you say your affirmations and you feel any doubt or negative feelings, immediately say them again and this time with all the positive belief that you can muster.

If you find it difficult to remember your affirmations, just jot them down on your 'to do' list, your shopping list or your diary. Then each time you see them, say them to yourself two or three times.

Affirmations are completely personal. No one needs to hear them or even know that you make them. The only rule is that they just have to be what you want, such as:

- I deserve more money.

- I am going to get a better job.

- I am great.

- I am fun to be with.

- I am going to ask him/her out.

- I will tell him/her that I don't agree.

- I will have more time for myself.

- I won't let them get to me.

- I am successful in everything I do.

Visualisations are very like affirmations, but you make mental pictures of whatever you want to happen. You need to create a clear picture of the object, person or situation in the way that you want it to be. Make the picture in the present and not the future: this way you can see things happening rather than waiting for them to happen. Include as many details as you can so that the image is as real as possible. As with affirmations, you should bring this picture to mind as often as you can, keeping the thoughts that surround the picture positive and full of energy.

Visualisation should be a pleasant, uplifting process – not exhausting, or you will defeat the object. The more you visualise your situation, the more it becomes part of your life and closer to reality.

Affirmations and visualisations are ways to think and see yourself reaching your goals and achieving your own success in a personal way. When you have been doing them for a while you will notice subtle changes, and your friends and colleagues will keep saying how much more positive and 'up' you seem.

Relaxation

If you are fit and healthy and detoxed, relaxation can be a continual state. That is not to say that you will be so relaxed that you never do anything or you stop responding to outside stimuli. Rather, that everything you do is done in a way that does not harm your body or put you under any unnecessary stress. You can be making a presentation to 500 delegates at a conference but still remain relaxed, and you can stand in a queue at the supermarket with four impatient children and still remain relaxed. All you have to do is use some simple relaxation techniques.

Once you have combined affirmations and visualisations (see page 90) and correct breathing (see page 87), it is very easy to keep yourself in a permanent state of relaxation. This is not a permanent state of being 'laid-back' or 'not caring', but a permanent state of being in control, calm and confident.

We have discussed breathing and what an important part it plays in staying relaxed. We have discussed visualisations and affirmations and how these can boost your confidence in achieving your goals. If you truly believe that you will get everything you want in life and you are 'centred and grounded' with regular deep breathing, then you will achieve true relaxation. Of course there are hurdles and hiccups along the way, but if you are confident about what the future holds for you, then relaxation is natural.

A simple relaxation exercise

Practice makes perfect. The more you actively practise relaxation techniques the more easy they become and, as with the breathing exercises, you will soon be able to take yourself into deep relaxation at any time during the day or night. All you have to do is memorise this sequence or even record it onto a tape and play it to yourself as you are relaxing.

1. Find a quiet room, make sure you are warm, and choose some music that is melodic and peaceful.

2. Lie down on the floor or sit comfortably in a chair.

3. Close your eyes and start to breathe deeply, as described in the breathing exercise on page 88.

4. After breathing correctly for a couple of minutes you should find that your breathing has slowed down and it should now feel very natural.

5. When you inhale, imagine that the air you are breathing is warm and golden and is bathing your body in warm, golden, restful and positive light.

6. Now start to consider how your body is feeling. As you inhale, start thinking about the feet and ankle areas of your body. Are they tense? If so, relax them.

7. As you exhale, picture the air you breathe out to be the old, stagnant air and the air you breathe in to be the new, fresh air.

8. Think of your calves and knees. Picture the warm air travelling through any tense muscles, bathing them in light. Exhale the stale air.

9. Picture your knee joints and your upper leg area. Breathe deeply and relax.

10. Feel the air being breathed into the groin area, relaxing the tension and soothing the pelvis. Breathe out the bad air.

11. See the golden light swirling around your stomach and abdomen, cleansing and uplifting your centre of emotion and spirit.

12. Watch the light thread its way between each and every rib, filling your lungs and chest cavity with warm, expanding air.

13. Watch each and every finger fill with golden light that spreads through your fingers and lower arms.

14. Breathe in the energy into your shoulders and base of your neck. Feel your neck relax and melt into the floor or back of the chair and up into the base of your skull.

15. The light may now travel into the root of each and every hair follicle, making your scalp feel invigorated and tingling.

16. Each time you exhale you are breathing out waste. Each time you breathe in you are breathing in new life.

17. When you have renewed the life inside your body, look to see where the source of your new breath and new light is coming from.

18. With your eyes still closed, look above you and see the beam of light coming down towards your

body – see it feeding into your abdomen. You are connected to this light and you can take as much as you wish.

19. Breathe deeply and inhale all you need.

20. When you are ready you can start to think about bringing your consciousness back into your own body and into the room you are in.

21. Open your eyes slowly. If you are lying on the floor or bed, roll over onto your side and wait a few moments before pushing yourself up to a sitting and then a standing position.

22. You should now feel totally relaxed and invigorated – well done!

EXFOLIATION

Exfoliation

Exfoliation is a very effective way to promote your Detox Programme. With all the benefits of the brushing technique, exfoliation can be included in the more relaxing, more tranquil or even indulgent times of the Detox Programme. This process is generally more gentle on the skin than dry brushing and can therefore be used both on the body and on the face and any other delicate areas that might find dry brushing a little too harsh. The idea of exfoliating is to scrub away dry skin, but if the product you are using is wet or oily it will not get rid of dry skin efficiently, but simply stimulate circulation.

There are many exfoliating products on the market, but I recommend the dry varieties for the optimum benefits. Whichever style product you choose, just make sure you carry it out once every three days while on the programme. Exfoliation needs some form of home-made or shop/salon-bought exfoliant products, which are widely available in all price ranges and are usually combined with wonderful-smelling essential oils.

You can exfoliate at any time of the day, but as I now recommend a dry exfoliator, it is definitely best or more convenient if you are standing in the bath, in the shower or on a towel to catch the grinds of the exfoliant and your dead skin (yuk!).

Either standing or sitting in an empty bath or shower, take very small amounts of the chosen scrub and press firmly against your skin, keeping your hand flat to the skin so as to prevent all the exfoliant from falling away, move in firm, stimulating, circular movements around the body. When the grinds run out, just scoop up a little more. It is surprising how the natural oils of your hands and body skin will keep much of the granules stuck in your palm to make the scrubbing more stimulating and effective. Pay special attention to any areas of hard skin – heels, knees, elbows and so on – and rub as hard as you find comfortable. The whole process should take about three or four minutes. When you have completed the rub, turn on the bath taps or shower and wash the residue off, the fragrance should stay but the salts wash away. Get out of the bath or shower and then rub yourself dry with a towel (not one that has been rinsed in fabric conditioner, as this will increase its absorbency and carry on the exfoliating process as you are drying yourself). Once you are dry, apply a good moisturiser or body oil all over your body and stay warm. Going to bed with a book or for an early night is a good next move.

Normally, the exfoliant you choose for your body would be too harsh for your face, so complete the process by changing over to the facial exfoliant and get your face glowing with health as well.

Now that you are aware of all the body-care treatments that are a required part of the Detox Programme you can plan the timing of your own programme and decide exactly when to start. Over the following pages there is a chart to complete for every day of the programme. Make sure that you tick each box every day, and then you can be sure that nothing has been missed. You may want to photocopy the chart before you begin.

Daily food and activity checklist

	1	2	3	4	5	6	7	8
Cold shower/bath	☐	☐	☐	☐	☐	☐	☐	☐
Dry-skin brushing	☐	☐	☐	☐	☐	☐	☐	☐
Moisturising	☐	☐	☐	☐	☐	☐	☐	☐
Hot lemon and water	☐	☐	☐	☐	☐	☐	☐	☐
Fruit	☐	☐	☐	☐	☐	☐	☐	☐
Goat's/sheep's yogurt	☐	☐	☐	☐	☐	☐	☐	☐
Goat's/sheep's cheese	☐	☐	☐	☐	☐	☐	☐	☐
Nuts	☐	☐	☐	☐	☐	☐	☐	☐
Seeds/pulses/beans	☐	☐	☐	☐	☐	☐	☐	☐
Brown rice	☐	☐	☐	☐	☐	☐	☐	☐
Salads	☐	☐	☐	☐	☐	☐	☐	☐
Fish (optional)	☐	☐	☐	☐	☐	☐	☐	☐
1.5 litres (2¾ pints) of water	☐	☐	☐	☐	☐	☐	☐	☐
Herbal teas	☐	☐	☐	☐	☐	☐	☐	☐
A good selection of superfoods	☐	☐	☐	☐	☐	☐	☐	☐
20 minutes' exercise	☐	☐	☐	☐	☐	☐	☐	☐
10 minutes' total relaxation	☐	☐	☐	☐	☐	☐	☐	☐
5 minutes' 'quality' breathing	☐	☐	☐	☐	☐	☐	☐	☐
5 affirmations or visualisations repeated 10 times each	☐	☐	☐	☐	☐	☐	☐	☐
Smile or laugh heartily	☐	☐	☐	☐	☐	☐	☐	☐
Exfoliation every third day	☐	☐	☐	☐	☐	☐	☐	☐
Treatment every 4 days: aromatherapy, massage, reflexology, etc. (optional)	☐	☐	☐	☐	☐	☐	☐	☐

Daily food and activity checklist

	9	10	11	12	13	14	15	16
Cold shower/bath	☐	☐	☐	☐	☐	☐	☐	☐
Dry-skin brushing	☐	☐	☐	☐	☐	☐	☐	☐
Moisturising	☐	☐	☐	☐	☐	☐	☐	☐
Hot lemon and water	☐	☐	☐	☐	☐	☐	☐	☐
Fruit	☐	☐	☐	☐	☐	☐	☐	☐
Goat's/sheep's yogurt	☐	☐	☐	☐	☐	☐	☐	☐
Goat's/sheep's cheese	☐	☐	☐	☐	☐	☐	☐	☐
Nuts	☐	☐	☐	☐	☐	☐	☐	☐
Seeds/pulses/beans	☐	☐	☐	☐	☐	☐	☐	☐
Brown rice	☐	☐	☐	☐	☐	☐	☐	☐
Salads	☐	☐	☐	☐	☐	☐	☐	☐
Fish (optional)	☐	☐	☐	☐	☐	☐	☐	☐
1.5 litres (2¾ pints) of water	☐	☐	☐	☐	☐	☐	☐	☐
Herbal teas	☐	☐	☐	☐	☐	☐	☐	☐
A good selection of superfoods	☐	☐	☐	☐	☐	☐	☐	☐
20 minutes' exercise	☐	☐	☐	☐	☐	☐	☐	☐
10 minutes' total relaxation	☐	☐	☐	☐	☐	☐	☐	☐
5 minutes' 'quality' breathing	☐	☐	☐	☐	☐	☐	☐	☐
5 affirmations or visualisations repeated 10 times each	☐	☐	☐	☐	☐	☐	☐	☐
Smile or laugh heartily	☐	☐	☐	☐	☐	☐	☐	☐
Exfoliation every third day	☐	☐	☐	☐	☐	☐	☐	☐
Treatment every 4 days: aromatherapy, massage, reflexology, etc. (optional)	☐	☐	☐	☐	☐	☐	☐	☐

Daily food and activity checklist

	17	18	19	20	21	22	23	24
Cold shower/bath	☐	☐	☐	☐	☐	☐	☐	☐
Dry-skin brushing	☐	☐	☐	☐	☐	☐	☐	☐
Moisturising	☐	☐	☐	☐	☐	☐	☐	☐
Hot lemon and water	☐	☐	☐	☐	☐	☐	☐	☐
Fruit	☐	☐	☐	☐	☐	☐	☐	☐
Goat's/sheep's yogurt	☐	☐	☐	☐	☐	☐	☐	☐
Goat's/sheep's cheese	☐	☐	☐	☐	☐	☐	☐	☐
Nuts	☐	☐	☐	☐	☐	☐	☐	☐
Seeds/pulses/beans	☐	☐	☐	☐	☐	☐	☐	☐
Brown rice	☐	☐	☐	☐	☐	☐	☐	☐
Salads	☐	☐	☐	☐	☐	☐	☐	☐
Fish (optional)	☐	☐	☐	☐	☐	☐	☐	☐
1.5 litres (2³/₄ pints) of water	☐	☐	☐	☐	☐	☐	☐	☐
Herbal teas	☐	☐	☐	☐	☐	☐	☐	☐
A good selection of superfoods	☐	☐	☐	☐	☐	☐	☐	☐
20 minutes' exercise	☐	☐	☐	☐	☐	☐	☐	☐
10 minutes' total relaxation	☐	☐	☐	☐	☐	☐	☐	☐
5 minutes' 'quality' breathing	☐	☐	☐	☐	☐	☐	☐	☐
5 affirmations or visualisations repeated 10 times each	☐	☐	☐	☐	☐	☐	☐	☐
Smile or laugh heartily	☐	☐	☐	☐	☐	☐	☐	☐
Exfoliation every third day	☐	☐	☐	☐	☐	☐	☐	☐
Treatment every 4 days: aromatherapy, massage, reflexology, etc. (optional)	☐	☐	☐	☐	☐	☐	☐	☐

Daily food and activity checklist

	25	26	27	28	29	30
Cold shower/bath	☐	☐	☐	☐	☐	☐
Dry-skin brushing	☐	☐	☐	☐	☐	☐
Moisturising	☐	☐	☐	☐	☐	☐
Hot lemon and water	☐	☐	☐	☐	☐	☐
Fruit	☐	☐	☐	☐	☐	☐
Goat's/sheep's yogurt	☐	☐	☐	☐	☐	☐
Goat's/sheep's cheese	☐	☐	☐	☐	☐	☐
Nuts	☐	☐	☐	☐	☐	☐
Seeds/pulses/beans	☐	☐	☐	☐	☐	☐
Brown rice	☐	☐	☐	☐	☐	☐
Salads	☐	☐	☐	☐	☐	☐
Fish (optional)	☐	☐	☐	☐	☐	☐
1.5 litres (2¾ pints) of water	☐	☐	☐	☐	☐	☐
Herbal teas	☐	☐	☐	☐	☐	☐
A good selection of superfoods	☐	☐	☐	☐	☐	☐
20 minutes' exercise	☐	☐	☐	☐	☐	☐
10 minutes' total relaxation	☐	☐	☐	☐	☐	☐
5 minutes' 'quality' breathing	☐	☐	☐	☐	☐	☐
5 affirmations or visualisations repeated 10 times each	☐	☐	☐	☐	☐	☐
Smile or laugh heartily	☐	☐	☐	☐	☐	☐
Exfoliation every third day	☐	☐	☐	☐	☐	☐
Treatment every 4 days: aromatherapy, massage, reflexology, etc. (optional)	☐	☐	☐	☐	☐	☐

The 30-day programme – trouble-shooting and common side effects

Problem/condition	Reason/solution
Fuzzy tongue/bad breath	This is a normal sign that the body is getting rid of toxins. Rinse your mouth each morning with lemon water or scrape your tongue with a toothbrush until it feels cleaner. During the day you can chew on parsley if you find that the garlic is affecting your breath.
Headache	Detoxing means you will be 'coming off' some chemicals such as caffeine, alcohol or sugar. This may cause mild headaches as your body adjusts and is quite normal. Drinking fluids, taking rest and relaxation will help relieve the discomfort.
Constipation	Change in diet may sometimes lead to mild constipation. This should not last for more than a few days. Eat plenty of rice and raw vegetables and check that you are not eating too much cheese. You will soon find your bowel movements becoming healthy and regular.
Tiredness/lethargy	When your body first embarks on the detox it will be hard work on the internal organs and can, although not always, be tiring. This will last for only a few days as you go through your 'healing crisis', and after that you will feel very energetic. If you feel tired later on during the programme you should check that you are eating enough – too little food can be very draining.
Flu-like symptoms	Again, these can be due to the expected starting 'changes' during the programme

Problem/condition	Reason/solution
	and are normal in the first week or so. If you feel any of these symptoms after the first ten days look at the quantities you are eating and check that they are enough. Also look at how much you are exercising – you may be doing too much too soon.
Loose bowels	During the first three weeks of the programme your bowel movements will be loose. This is a result of the increased intake of fibre, the rice and the body cleaning out all its waste. This is normal and shows that the detox is working.
Nausea	This is not common and should be treated with caution. If you feel nauseous check you are eating enough and that your fluid intake is sufficient. Rest and relax, and don't exercise for that day.
Irritability	This is common. Try to do some breathing exercises or some actual exercise. Your body is going through some major changes and you should try to accommodate them as much as possible. It is just an indication that the bad is being cleared out!
Increased bowel movements	As with loose bowel movements, this is quite normal during detox. It is likely that you will be making at least two movements a day – a sign that your body is processing foods efficiently and effectively.
Coloured urine	When you take vitamin supplements your urine is likely to change to a bright yellow/orange colour, and when you drink freshly juiced fruit or vegetables your urine will also change colour depending on the fruit or vegetable chosen – beetroot will turn it pink!

Problem/condition	Reason/solution
Spots	The skin is the body's biggest organ of elimination, so spots are very common during detox. You can reduce the risk of them if you drink lots of fluid and plenty of herbal teas that are diuretic (make you pass water), such as dandelion or fennel.
Change in skin tone	The efficiency of your circulation is greatly increased during the detox programme. This can lead to temporary 'rosy cheeks' or a 'glow', which will settle as your body adapts to the programme.
Runny nose or eyes, or sinus congestion	During the early stages of the programme it is likely that you may experience a slightly runny or blocked nose. This simply indicates that your body is clearing out or balancing your own fluid production, and the symptoms will only last a couple of days at most.

5

Recipes and Eating Suggestions

There are so many foods available to you when detoxing that it would be near impossible to put them all in recipes for you to try. But try we have! Working with cookery writer Anne Sheasby, we have managed to transform what looks like an ordinary list of foods into some sumptuous feasts, delicious snacks and delightful desserts – there really is no reason not to eat like a king on your Detox Programme.

If you are not a recipe person and like to 'free form' in the kitchen, then just remember to use your imagination and to experiment – there will be meals that you make and choose not to do again, but there will also be meals that you create that will become a staple part of your eating programme long after you have finished the detox – send me any recipes you think are brilliant discoveries and you may see them in the next book or on my website: jane@janescrivner.com.

All the recipes in this chapter serve two, unless otherwise stated. Salt should not be added to any of the recipes; the natural salt contents of the foods should suffice. Cooking times are approximate; please refer to your manufacturer's guidelines for more specific information on adjusting the temperature or cooking period if applicable. Stay safe in your kitchen and enjoy the food – that's the legal bit out of the way.

The recipes and eating suggestions in this chapter are broken down into:

- Breakfasts

- Snacks

- Light meals, salads and side dishes

- Hearty soups

- Main courses

- Desserts

- Entertaining on the Detox Programme

- Logistical problems you may encounter while eating out on the Detox Programme, and solutions.

BREAKFASTS

HOME-MADE MUESLI

Preparation time: 5 minutes
Cooking time: N/A
Serves 2

Porridge oats (choose toasted oats, if desired)
Sunflower seeds
Sesame seeds
Pumpkin seeds
Ready-to-eat dried apricots, chopped
Natural sheep's yoghurt

1. In a bowl, mix together the oats, mixed seeds and chopped apricots. (You can vary the quantities and proportions of ingredients to suit your taste.)

2. Spoon or pour some yoghurt into two cereal bowls and sprinkle some oat and seed mixture over the top of each portion.

3. Serve the muesli as it is or stir gently before serving.

Variations

• Other dried fruits such as figs, pears, sultanas, raisins, cranberries, blueberries, or a mixture, may be substituted for the dried apricots.

• Top the muesli with a drizzle of runny (clear) honey, just before serving.

This recipe is suitable for vegetarians.

BLUEBERRY PORRIDGE WITH MIXED SEEDS

Piping hot porridge, drizzled with honey, sprinkled with mixed seeds and topped with fresh blueberries, provides a great start to the day and is ideal for a warming breakfast or brunch.

Preparation time: 10 minutes
Cooking time: 10 minutes
Serves 2

55g (2oz) porridge oats
400ml (14fl oz) water

A little honey, to taste (optional)
1 tablespoon pumpkin seeds, or to taste
1 tablespoon sunflower seeds, or to taste
200g (7oz) fresh blueberries, rinsed and patted dry

1. Place the oats in a non-stick saucepan and stir in the water. Bring gently to the boil, stirring, then simmer for about 5 minutes or until the desired consistency is achieved, stirring occasionally. Remove from the heat and leave to stand for 1–2 minutes before serving.

2. Spoon the porridge into two serving bowls and drizzle with a little honey, if desired. Sprinkle with the mixed seeds, scatter the blueberries over the top and serve.

Variations

• Lightly crush the seeds using a pestle and mortar.

• Fresh raspberries or strawberries may be substituted for the blueberries.

Cook's Tip

• Porridge can also be made in a microwave oven – simply follow the guidelines on the packet or follow the manufacturer's instructions.

This recipe is suitable for vegetarians.

Fresh fruit salad

Preparation time: 15 minutes
Cooking time: N/A
Serves 2

A mixture of your favourite fresh fruits (such as pears, apples, pineapple, grapes, melon and kiwi), prepared and chopped into bite-size cubes
Fresh unsweetened apple juice
Juice of 1 lime

1. Place the chopped fruit in a bowl and add enough apple juice to just cover the fruit.

2. Pour the lime juice over the top and stir lightly to mix. Spoon into serving bowls and serve.

Variations

- Use freshly squeezed lemon juice in place of lime juice.
- Freshly squeezed orange juice or fresh unsweetened pineapple juice may be substituted for the apple juice.

This recipe is suitable for vegetarians.

SNACKS

While you are on the Detox Programme you should never be really hungry – if you are, either you are not eating enough or you have left a long time between meals. Remember that five smaller meals a day are better than three big meals, the smaller meals will ensure you don't feel hungry but more importantly, you keep your energy levels steady and your metabolism regulated. Whatever your eating habits on the programme, there will always be times when you might like a light snack between meals. Obviously any of the dishes below can be made in smaller quantities, or you can eat any of the ingredients individually. Here are some other ideas for snacks.

POPCORN

Buy a packet as usual, but instead of making your popcorn in butter substitute olive oil. When the corn is ready you can add further flavour by tossing the warm kernels in a mixture of herbs.

RICE CAKES

These should be in the larder at home as an emergency snack. Make sure you buy the non-salted version, and have a selection of plain and sesame seed cakes to vary the flavour.

NUTS AND SEEDS

Make up a bag of mixed nuts and seeds to taste; you can also add chopped dried fruit for a little extra flavour. These are great, as they are small and will last in your handbag or desk for at least a week.

CRUDITÉS

A fairly posh name for chopped-up vegetables or salads to crunch away on or dip into the hummus or guacamole, or even just sesame seeds for a nutty taste sensation. Simply slice into bite-size pieces, carrots, celery, peppers, cauliflower florets, broccoli florets or anything that takes your fancy.

HUMMUS

Preparation time: 10 minutes (plus extra time for preparing the dried chickpeas, if necessary)
Cooking time: N/A
Serves 2

115g (4oz) tahini (light or dark)
Juice of 2 lemons
2–3 cloves garlic, crushed, or to taste
100ml (3½fl oz) olive oil
175g (6oz) dried chickpeas, soaked, cooked until tender (about 1–1½ hours) and drained, or 400g (14oz) can chickpeas, rinsed well and drained
Freshly ground black pepper, to taste
Chopped fresh parsley, to garnish (optional)

1. Put the tahini, lemon juice, garlic and olive oil in a blender or food processor and blend until smooth and well mixed.

2. Add the chickpeas and blend until a thick paste is formed. You can add a little water to loosen the consistency, a little extra olive oil to make it more creamy, or add more garlic and lemon juice to suit your taste. Season to taste with black pepper.

3. Spoon into a serving bowl and garnish with chopped parsley, if desired. Serve with a selection of fresh vegetable crudités, or keep in a covered container in the fridge and pack up for a portable snack.

This recipe is suitable for vegetarians.

MEXICAN AVOCADO DIP

Serve this tasty guacamole-style Mexican dip with a selection of fresh vegetable crudités, for a nutritious snack.

Preparation time: 10 minutes
Cooking time: N/A
Serves 2

2 ripe avocados
2 teaspoons lemon or lime juice, or to taste
1 spring onion, finely chopped
1 vine-ripened tomato, skinned, seeded and finely chopped
½ fresh red or green chilli, seeded and finely chopped (optional)
1 small clove garlic, crushed
2–3 teaspoons chopped fresh coriander
Freshly ground black pepper, to taste

1. Peel and stone the avocado, then mash the flesh in a bowl with the lemon or lime juice. Stir in the spring onion, tomato, chilli, if using, garlic and coriander and season to taste with black pepper.

2. Spoon the mixture into a serving bowl and serve immediately with a selection of fresh vegetable crudités such as carrot, cucumber and pepper sticks, cauliflower and broccoli florets and cherry tomatoes.

Cook's Tip

- Wear disposable gloves when preparing fresh chillies, as the natural oils in chillies may cause irritation to your skin and eyes. If you don't have any disposable gloves, make sure you wash your hands thoroughly after preparing the chilli.

This recipe is suitable for vegetarians.

PRAWN & BROCCOLI STIR-FRY

This is a quick and nutritious detox stir-fry, ideal for a tasty snack or light lunch.

Preparation time: 10 minutes
Cooking time: 8 minutes
Serves 2

1 tablespoon olive or sesame oil
1 red or yellow pepper, seeded and thinly sliced
1 small fresh red or green chilli, seeded and finely chopped (optional)
1cm (½in) piece fresh root ginger, peeled and finely chopped
1 clove garlic, finely chopped
175g (6oz) small broccoli florets
4 spring onions, chopped
115–140g (4–5oz) cooked peeled king prawns
4–6 tablespoons vegetable stock
2–3 teaspoons toasted sesame seeds (optional)
Freshly ground black pepper, to taste

1. Heat the olive or sesame oil in a wok or large frying pan. Add the pepper, chilli, if using, ginger, garlic, broccoli and spring onions and stir-fry over a fairly high heat for 3–5 minutes.

2. Add the prawns, stock and sesame seeds, if using, and stir-fry for 1–2 minutes, or until the prawns are hot. Season to taste with black pepper and serve immediately on its own or with cooked rice.

Variations

- Use fresh salmon fillets or tuna steaks, cut into thin strips, in place of the prawns. Add with the stock and stir-fry for 2–3 minutes or until cooked.
- Green beans (cut into short lengths) or courgettes (sliced) may be substituted for the broccoli.

Cook's Tip

- This recipe will serve one as a main course (with rice) or as a lunch or supper. To serve two as a main course, lunch or supper, simply double all the ingredient quantities given above (you may also need to increase the cooking time slightly).

LIGHT MEALS, SALADS AND SIDE DISHES

All the following recipes are suitable for everyday meals, salads or side dishes. They are quite simple and straightforward, but very tasty. It is a good idea to cook enough rice for two or three meals rather than each time you eat, as this will save time on preparation.

When oily fish such as tuna, mackerel or sardines are listed use fresh where possible, but canned versions are acceptable if they are in olive oil, vegetable oil or spring water. Try to avoid canned fish in brine, however, as the salt content is far too high. Remember: fresh is best.

When fruit or vegetables are listed, you must only use fresh produce. If it is not in season choose an available alternative to suit your taste – there really is no excuse for canned fruit or vegetables except canned tomatoes, and they are actually a bit more nutritious than when raw due to their high concentration.

But each meal must be a plate or bowl *full*, so don't restrict your portion size. As the food is all fresh it will generally keep until the next meal without dressings, so make more rather than less – you should not be hungry on the Detox Programme.

GREEK BAKED POTATOES

Preparation time: 10 minutes
Cooking time: 1½ hours, plus 10 minutes grilling time
Serves 2

2 large baking potatoes
115g (4oz) cucumber, diced
115g (4oz) ewe's feta cheese, diced
4 teaspoons sesame oil
2–3 tablespoons shredded fresh basil leaves
Freshly ground black pepper, to taste

1. Preheat the oven to 200°C/fan 180°C/gas mark 6. Wash and dry the potatoes, then prick them all over with a fork or wrap them in foil.

2. Place on a baking sheet (or directly on the oven shelf, if wrapped in foil) and bake in the oven for about 1½ hours or until the potatoes are cooked and feel soft when gently squeezed. Turn them over once during cooking. If you have foil-wrapped the potatoes, open up the foil after about 1 hour of the cooking time to allow the skins to crisp up.

3. Meanwhile, mix the cucumber and feta cheese together in a bowl and set aside. Preheat the grill to high. When the potatoes are ready, split them open and fork the sesame oil, basil and black pepper into the flesh. Push the flesh back into the skins and spoon the cucumber/feta mixture over the top.

4. Place the potatoes in a flameproof dish and heat under the grill until the feta begins to melt. Serve with a side salad of mixed lettuce leaves, accompanied by a *small* glass of mineral water.

This recipe is suitable for vegetarians.

CHILLI-SPICED COURGETTE GRILL WITH RICE

Preparation time: 10 minutes (plus extra time for cooking the rice)
Cooking time: 10 minutes
Serves 2

Long-grain brown rice, cooked, drained and kept hot (allow about 85g/3oz *raw* weight per serving)

2 large courgettes, sliced
1 red pepper, seeded and sliced
1 green pepper, seeded and sliced
115g (4oz) ewe's feta cheese, sliced
Chilli powder (mild or hot), to taste

1. Preheat the grill to medium. Put the cooked hot rice in the bottom of a heatproof bowl or flameproof dish, set aside and keep hot.

2. Place the courgette slices in steamer over a pan of boiling water for a few minutes or until tender but still crunchy. Drain well

3. Mix the courgettes and peppers together, then spoon this mixture over the hot rice. Arrange the feta slices on top.

4. Place the dish under the grill until the cheese has lightly browned on top. Sprinkle with chilli powder to taste and serve.

This recipe is suitable for vegetarians.

CRUNCHY RED COLESLAW WITH FLAKED MACKEREL

Preparation time: 15 minutes
Cooking time: N/A
Serves 2

8 radishes, chopped
1 red pepper, seeded and thinly sliced
1/2 cucumber, cut into thin strips
2 carrots, grated
1/2 small red cabbage, thinly shredded

1–2 tablespoons extra-virgin olive oil
4 teaspoons freshly squeezed lime juice
Freshly ground black pepper, to taste
2 smoked mackerel fillets, each about 85–100g (3–3½oz)
2 tablespoons chopped fresh coriander

1. Mix all the prepared vegetables together in a bowl. In a separate small bowl, whisk together the olive oil and lime juice and season to taste with black pepper. Drizzle the dressing over the vegetables and toss lightly to mix.

2. Divide the coleslaw between two serving plates or soup bowls. Flake the mackerel fillets and lay the flakes on top of the coleslaw, then sprinkle the fish with chopped coriander. Serve with a *small* glass of fresh unsweetened apple juice.

Variations

- Flaked smoked trout may be substituted for the smoked mackerel.
- Use one yellow or orange pepper in place of the red pepper.

Cook's Tip

The quantities of vegetables given above are a guide only so vary the quantities according to taste, and add a little extra dressing, if desired.

BEETROOT & FENNEL SALAD WITH MIXED NUTS

Preparation time: 15 minutes
Cooking time: N/A
Serves 2

4 tablespoons cashew nuts, roughly chopped
4 tablespoons pine nuts
2 beetroot, cooked and chopped
1 fennel bulb, chopped or thinly sliced
About 85g (3oz) lettuce, shredded
½ cucumber, chopped
1 green pepper, seeded and chopped
4–6 tablespoons nut or seed oil (such as walnut, hazelnut, sesame or
   pumpkin seed oil) or extra-virgin olive oil
Juice of 1 lemon
4 tablespoons chopped fresh coriander
Freshly ground black pepper, to taste

1. Put the nuts and prepared vegetables in a bowl and toss
to mix. In a separate small bowl, whisk together the oil,
lemon juice and chopped coriander. Season to taste
with black pepper.

2. Drizzle the dressing over the salad and toss gently to
mix. Serve the dressed salad on its own or on top of a
bed of cooked (cold or hot) brown rice. Alternatively,
you can serve the salad as an accompaniment to any of
the main course dishes.

Variations

- Lightly toast the nuts before serving, to add a little extra flavour.

- Use hazelnuts in place of cashew nuts.

This recipe is suitable for vegetarians.

THREE-BEAN SALAD

Preparation time: 10 minutes (plus extra time for preparing the dried beans, if necessary)
Cooking time: N/A
Serves 2

85g (3oz) dried red kidney beans, soaked, cooked until tender and drained, *or* 225g (8oz) can red kidney beans, rinsed well and drained
85g (3oz) dried chickpeas, soaked, cooked until tender and drained, *or* 215g (7½oz) can chickpeas, rinsed well and drained
85g (3oz) dried butter beans, soaked, cooked until tender and drained, *or* 215g (7½oz) can butter beans, rinsed well and drained
1 red onion, thinly sliced
1 small red or yellow pepper, seeded and diced
85g (3oz) mangetout or sugar-snap peas, chopped
3–4 tablespoons extra-virgin olive oil
Juice of ½ lemon
1 clove garlic, crushed or finely chopped
1–2 tablespoons chopped fresh mixed herbs
Freshly ground black pepper, to taste

1. Put the cooked or canned beans in a bowl, add the onion, red or yellow pepper and mangetout or sugar-snap peas and toss to mix well.

2. In a separate small bowl, whisk together the oil, lemon juice, garlic and chopped herbs, then season to taste with black pepper.

3. Pour the dressing over the bean salad and toss to mix. Cover and leave in the fridge for at least 1 hour before serving, to allow the flavours to blend.

4. Serve the bean salad on its own or on a bed of mixed lettuce leaves or cooked (cold) brown rice. Serve with a *small* glass of mineral water or fresh unsweetened apple juice, if desired.

Variations

• Use 4–6 spring onions in place of the red onion.

• Use snipped fresh chives in place of mixed herbs.

Cook's Tip

Follow the general guidelines for bean soaking (usually overnight) and cooking on the packet or box, then drain and boil together until tender (about 1–1½ hours).

This recipe is suitable for vegetarians.

HEARTY SOUPS

I love hearty soups, no matter what time of the year it is. A bowl of warm soup is satisfying, tasty and simple to prepare. You can make larger amounts and freeze it or make it fresh every time, but having some in the freezer means you simply have to defrost and reheat it for a tasty ready meal – fast food the detox way.

Plum tomato, lentil & fresh basil soup

Lentils add lovely substance and texture to the classic aromatic combination of tomatoes and basil, to create this really satisfying, hearty soup.

Preparation time: 10 minutes
Cooking time: 30 minutes
Serves 2

55g (2oz) Puy lentils
1 tablespoon olive oil
1 red onion, chopped
400g (14oz) can plum tomatoes
450ml (16fl oz) vegetable stock
1 bay leaf
Freshly ground black pepper, to taste
2 tablespoons shredded fresh basil leaves
Small fresh basil sprigs, to garnish

1. Rinse the lentils, then add them to a pan of boiling water. Cover and simmer for about 15–20 minutes, or until tender. Drain well, rinse, then drain again and set aside.

2. Meanwhile, heat the olive oil in a separate saucepan, add the onion and sauté for about 5 minutes or until softened. Stir in the tomatoes and their juice, the stock and bay leaf and season with black pepper. Bring to the boil, then reduce the heat, cover and simmer for 20 minutes, stirring occasionally.

3. Remove the pan from the heat and cool slightly, then discard the bay leaf. Purée the soup using a hand-held (stick) blender (or in a blender or food processor), until smooth and combined. Stir in the cooked lentils and shredded basil and gently reheat the soup until hot, stirring. Ladle into warmed soup bowls, garnish with basil sprigs and serve.

Variations

• A standard (white) onion or 3 shallots may be substituted for the red onion, if desired.

• Fresh tomatoes may be used in place of canned tomatoes. You will need about 500g (1lb 2oz) fresh plum or vine-ripened tomatoes, which you then need to skin, seed and chop before adding to the softened onion. You may also need to increase the quantity of stock a little.

Cook's Tip

• To save a little time, you could use about 140g (5oz) canned green lentils (well rinsed and drained) in place of the Puy lentils. Simply add the canned lentils with the shredded basil in the last stages of the recipe.

This recipe is suitable for vegetarians.

CUMIN-SPICED CARROT SOUP

This deliciously thick, spiced soup is ideal for warming up those cold autumn or winter evenings.

Preparation time: 10 minutes
Cooking time: 40 minutes
Serves 2

1 tablespoon olive oil
1 onion, chopped
1 clove garlic, crushed
1 stick celery, chopped
1½ teaspoons ground cumin, or to taste
350g (12oz) carrots (about 3–4 carrots), thinly sliced
600ml (1 pint) vegetable stock
Freshly ground black pepper, to taste
Chopped fresh coriander, to garnish (optional)

1. Heat the olive oil in a saucepan, add the onion, garlic and celery and sauté for about 5 minutes or until softened. Add the cumin and cook gently for 1 minute, stirring.

2. Stir in the carrots and stock and season with black pepper. Bring to the boil, then reduce the heat, cover and simmer for about 30 minutes, or until the carrots are tender, stirring occasionally.

3. Remove the pan from the heat and cool slightly, then purée the soup using a hand-held (stick) blender (or in a blender or food processor), until smooth and combined. Gently reheat the soup until hot, stirring. Ladle into warmed soup bowls, garnish with chopped coriander, if desired, and serve.

Variations

- Use 3 shallots in place of the onion.

- Ground coriander may be substituted for the cumin. Also stir a little chopped fresh coriander through the hot soup just before serving to enhance the coriander flavour even more.

- Use parsnips in place of the carrots and try using curry powder instead of cumin.

This recipe is suitable for vegetarians.

PEA & ONION SOUP

This tasty combination of vegetables creates a lovely warming soup, ideal for a satisfying lunch or supper.

Preparation time: 10 minutes
Cooking time: 20–25 minutes
Serves 2

1 tablespoon sunflower oil
1 small onion, finely chopped
1 leek, washed and thinly sliced
1 small baking potato (about 200g/7oz unprepared weight), peeled and diced
450ml (16fl oz) vegetable stock
Freshly ground black pepper, to taste
175g (6oz) fresh peas (shelled weight) or frozen peas
2 tablespoons chopped fresh parsley
Fresh parsley sprigs, to garnish (optional)

1. Heat the sunflower oil in a saucepan. Add the onion and leek and sauté for about 5 minutes or until softened. Stir in the potato and stock and season with black pepper. If you are using fresh peas, add them at this stage; if you are using frozen peas, add them in 10–15 minutes time.

2. Bring the mixture to the boil, then reduce the heat, cover and simmer for 15–20 minutes, or until the vegetables are tender, stirring occasionally.

3. Remove the pan from the heat and cool slightly, then purée the soup using a hand-held (stick) blender (or in a blender or food processor), until smooth and combined. Stir in the chopped parsley and gently reheat the soup until hot, stirring. Ladle into warmed soup bowls, garnish with parsley sprigs, if desired, and serve.

Variations

• 2–3 shallots may be substituted for the onion, if desired.

• Use snipped fresh chives or coriander in place of the parsley.

This recipe is suitable for vegetarians.

BUTTERNUT SQUASH & LEEK SOUP

This lovely, mildly spiced, warming vegetable soup creates a very tempting lunch or supper, ideal for detox days.

Preparation time: 15 minutes
Cooking time: 30–35 minutes
Serves 2

1 tablespoon olive oil
1 small onion or 2 shallots, chopped

2 small leeks, washed and thinly sliced (about 115g/4oz prepared
  weight)
1 clove garlic, crushed (optional)
1 teaspoon ground cumin
1 teaspoon ground coriander
225g (8oz) diced butternut squash (prepared/peeled and seeded
  weight – see Cook's Tips)
600ml (1 pint) vegetable stock
Freshly ground black pepper, to taste
Chopped fresh coriander, to garnish (optional)

1. Heat the olive oil in a saucepan, add the onion, leeks
and garlic, if using, and sauté for about 5 minutes or
until softened. Add the ground spices and cook gently
for 1 minute, stirring.

2. Stir in the squash and stock and season with black
pepper. Bring to the boil, then reduce the heat, cover
and simmer for 20–25 minutes, or until the vegetables
are tender, stirring occasionally.

3. Remove the pan from the heat and cool slightly, then
puree the soup using a hand-held (stick) blender (or in
a blender or food processor), until smooth and
combined. Gently reheat the soup until hot, stirring.
Ladle into warmed soup bowls, garnish with a sprinkling of chopped coriander, if desired, and serve.

Cook's Tips

- ½ butternut squash (whole weight about 700g/1lb 9oz)
  creates about 225g (8oz) prepared (peeled and seeded)
  flesh.

- For a stronger spicy flavour, increase the quantity of ground cumin and coriander to 1½–2 teaspoons of each. Alternatively, add a sprinkling of hot chilli powder with the other ground spices, to give a hot boost to the flavour.

This recipe is suitable for vegetarians.

FRESH MUSHROOM SOUP WITH PARSLEY

A simple, classic mushroom soup flavoured with fresh parsley and ideal for a tasty lunch or supper.

Preparation time: 10 minutes
Cooking time: 25–30 minutes
Serves 2

1 tablespoon sunflower oil
3 shallots, chopped
225g (8oz) mushrooms (chestnut or closed cup), sliced
600ml (1 pint) vegetable stock
Freshly ground black pepper, to taste
2–3 tablespoons chopped fresh parsley
Fresh parsley sprigs, to garnish (optional)

1. Heat the sunflower oil in a saucepan, add the shallots and sauté for about 5 minutes or until softened. Add the mushrooms and cook gently for 3 minutes, stirring occasionally.

2. Stir in the stock and season with black pepper. Bring to the boil, then reduce the heat, cover and simmer for 15–20 minutes or until the vegetables are tender, stirring occasionally.

3. Remove the pan from the heat and cool slightly, then purée the soup using a hand-held (stick) blender (or in a blender or food processor), until smooth and combined. Stir in the chopped parsley and gently reheat the soup until hot, stirring. Ladle into warmed soup bowls, garnish with parsley sprigs, if desired, and serve.

Variations

• Use 1 leek, washed and thinly sliced, or 1 onion, in place of the shallots.

• Snipped fresh chives may be substituted for the parsley.

Cook's Tip

• To add extra flavour to this soup, soak a few dried porcini mushrooms in a little boiling water for about 20 minutes. Strain the liquid and reserve. Chop the porcini. Add the chopped porcini with the fresh mushrooms and the porcini liquid with the stock in the recipe above.

This recipe is suitable for vegetarians.

MAIN COURSES

These dishes are slightly more complicated and will probably need thirty minutes' preparation. All of them would be very suitable for entertaining at home, and of course they are also great for something different for your own main meals.

Chargrilled salmon with watercress

Preparation time: 10 minutes
Cooking time: 8 minutes
Serves 2

2 salmon steaks or fillets, each about 115–175g (4–6oz)
115g (4oz) watercress
1/4 red cabbage, finely shredded
1 red onion, thinly sliced
20 pitted black olives
115g (4oz) ewe's feta cheese
Juice of 1 lime
2 tablespoons extra-virgin olive oil

1. Preheat the grill to medium. Place the salmon steaks or fillets on the rack in a grill pan and grill for about 4 minutes on each side or until slightly browned on top but just cooked and still moist in the centre, turning once.

2. Meanwhile, divide the watercress evenly between two serving plates, scatter the red cabbage over the watercress, then place the onion slices on top. Scatter the olives over the onion, then roughly crumble the cheese over the top.

3. Place the hot grilled salmon on top and dress with lime juice and olive oil. Serve with a *small* glass of fresh unsweetened apple juice.

Variations

- Fresh tuna steaks may be substituted for the salmon.

- Use the juice of 1 small lemon in place of the lime juice.

- Baby spinach or rocket leaves may be substituted for the watercress.

GRILLED COD & COLCANNON

Colcannon is a popular Scottish way of serving mashed potato. This is the detox version which leaves out the cream and butter but is just as tasty and far healthier!

Preparation time: 15 minutes
Cooking time: 20 minutes
Serves 2

3 large potatoes, peeled and diced
3–4 tablespoons olive oil, or to taste
2 small leeks, washed and finely shredded
115–175g (4–6oz) green cabbage (Savoy is best), finely shredded
2 cloves garlic, crushed
2 cod steaks or fillets, each about 115–175g (4–6oz)
1–2 tablespoons snipped fresh chives (optional)
Freshly ground black pepper, to taste

1. Preheat the grill to medium. Cook the potatoes in a pan of boiling water for 15–20 minutes or until cooked.

2. Meanwhile, heat 1–2 tablespoons of olive oil in a frying pan, add the leeks, cabbage and garlic and sauté until lightly browned.

3. In the meantime, lightly brush the cod steaks or fillets with a little oil, then place them on the rack in a grill pan. Grill the cod for about 4 minutes on each side or until cooked and lightly golden on top, turning once.

4. Drain, then mash the cooked potatoes with a little oil to loosen. Add the fried vegetables and snipped chives, if using, and stir together to roughly mix – the texture of the mashed potatoes will be quite rough once it has been mixed with the vegetables.

5. Pile the potato mixture onto the centre of two warmed serving plates and place a grilled cod steak or fillet on top of each portion. Sprinkle with black pepper and serve immediately with lightly cooked green vegetables such as broccoli, green beans or spinach.

Variations

- Other white fish such as haddock or halibut may be substituted for the cod.

- Use 1–2 bunches of spring onions, chopped, in place of the leeks.

SMOKED HADDOCK WITH PINE NUT & CORIANDER CRUMBLE

Preparation time: 10 minutes
Cooking time: 8–10 minutes
Serves 2

2 tablespoons pine nuts
2 tablespoons chopped fresh coriander

Freshly ground black pepper, to taste

About 4 teaspoons olive oil, plus extra for brushing and frying

2 fillets undyed smoked haddock, each about 175g (6oz)

2 courgettes, sliced

1 large onion, chopped

1. Preheat the grill to medium. Using a pestle and mortar, crush together 1 tablespoon of the pine nuts with the chopped coriander and some black pepper. Add enough olive oil drop by drop until you have a stiff paste, then stir in the remaining pine nuts (leaving them whole). Set aside.

2. Lightly brush the haddock fillets with a little oil, then place them on the rack in a grill pan. Grill for about 5–6 minutes or until cooked through, turning once.

3. Spread some of the pine nut and coriander mixture on top of each fish fillet, dividing it evenly, then continue to grill for a few more minutes until the crumble is lightly browned.

4. In the meantime, heat a little olive oil in a frying pan, add the courgettes and onion and sauté until just golden.

5. Spoon the courgette and onion mixture onto two warmed serving plates, then place the haddock fillets on top. Sprinkle with more black pepper and serve on its own or with a mixed dark leaf salad or lightly cooked green vegetables such as spinach or tenderstem broccoli.

FLAKED TUNA, CHICKPEA & CHERRY TOMATO SALAD

Canned or fresh tuna, chickpeas and cherry tomatoes combine well to create this tasty main-course salad.

Preparation time: 15 minutes
Cooking time: N/A
Serves 2

400g (14oz) can chickpeas
115g (4oz) cherry tomatoes, halved
1 small red pepper, seeded and diced
85g (3oz) sugar-snap peas or mangetout, chopped
85g (3oz) watercress or baby spinach leaves (or a mixture of water
  cress, baby spinach and rocket)
200g (7oz) can tuna in spring water, drained and flaked *or* 225g
  (8oz) fresh tuna steak, grilled, cooled and flaked
3 tablespoons extra-virgin olive oil
1½ teaspoons balsamic vinegar
2–3 teaspoons chopped fresh mixed herbs
Freshly ground black pepper, to taste

1. Rinse the chickpeas well, then drain and put them in a bowl. Add the cherry tomatoes, red pepper, sugar-snap peas or mangetout, watercress or spinach and flaked tuna and toss.

2. Put the olive oil, vinegar and chopped herbs in a small bowl and whisk together. Season to taste with black pepper. Drizzle the dressing over the salad and toss gently to mix, then serve.

Variations

- Use canned flageolet or black-eye beans in place of chickpeas.

- Canned or grilled fresh salmon or mackerel fillets may be substituted for the tuna, if desired.

Cook's Tip

- To make this salad into a quick and tasty snack for two, simply halve the ingredient quantities given in the recipe above.

SALADE NIÇOISE

Preparation time: 15 minutes, plus 2 hours marinating time
Cooking time: 15 minutes
Serves 2

3–4 tablespoons olive oil
Juice of 1 lemon
1–2 tablespoons chopped fresh mixed herbs
2 fresh tuna steaks, each about 140g (5oz)
280–350g (10–12oz) baby new potatoes
115g (4oz) green or French beans, cut in half
1–2 cloves garlic, finely chopped
1–2 tablespoons chopped fresh coriander
Freshly ground black pepper, to taste
2 tablespoons pine nuts, toasted
Two good handfuls of mixed lettuce leaves
20 pitted black olives, halved

1. In a shallow non-metallic dish, whisk together 2 tablespoons of the olive oil, half of the lemon juice and all the chopped herbs. Add the tuna steaks to the dish and turn them in the marinade to coat all over. Cover and leave to marinate in the fridge for a couple of hours.

2. Cook the potatoes in a pan of boiling water for 10–15 minutes, or until tender. Add the green beans to the potatoes about 4–5 minutes before the end of the cooking time. Drain thoroughly and keep warm.

3. Meanwhile, preheat the grill to medium. Remove the tuna steaks from the marinade (discard the marinade) and place them on the rack in a grill pan. Grill for 4–5 minutes on each side or until cooked through and lightly golden, turning once.

4. In a small bowl, whisk together the remaining olive oil and lemon juice, the garlic and chopped coriander and season to taste with black pepper. Stir in the pine nuts.

5. Put the warm potatoes and green beans, lettuce and olives in a large bowl and toss to mix. Pile the mixture onto two warmed serving plates, then place a grilled tuna steak on top of each portion. Drizzle the pine nut dressing over the tuna and salad, and serve.

OVEN-BAKED STUFFED PEPPERS WITH CUCUMBER SALAD

Preparation time: 15 minutes (plus extra time for cooking the rice)
Cooking time: 30 minutes
Serves 2

2 large red peppers
200g (7oz) soft or creamy goat's cheese
2–3 tablespoons shredded fresh basil leaves

2 cloves garlic, thinly sliced
Long-grain brown rice, cooked, drained and kept hot (allow about
  55–85g/2– 3oz *raw* weight per serving)
4 tablespoons extra-virgin olive oil, plus extra for drizzling
About 115g (4oz) assorted lettuce leaves
1/2 cucumber, thinly sliced
Juice of 1 small lemon
Freshly ground black pepper, to taste
Sesame seeds (toasted, if preferred), to sprinkle

1. Preheat the oven to 180°C/fan 160°C/gas mark 4. Slice each red pepper in half vertically, remove the cores and seeds, then place the pepper halves, cut side up, on a baking sheet. Bake in the oven for about 10 minutes or until they are beginning to soften.

2. Meanwhile, mix together the cheese, basil, garlic and rice in a bowl. Remove the pepper halves from the oven and spoon some rice mixture into each pepper half, piling it up if necessary and dividing it evenly. Drizzle a little olive oil over each stuffed pepper half, then return them to the oven and bake for a further 20 minutes or until cooked.

3. In the meantime, in a salad bowl, mix together the lettuce leaves and cucumber. In a separate small bowl, whisk together the 4 tablespoons of olive oil and the lemon juice and season to taste with black pepper. Drizzle the dressing over the salad and toss lightly to mix. Sprinkle the salad with sesame seeds. Serve the hot stuffed peppers with the cucumber salad alongside.

This recipe is suitable for vegetarians.

ROAST GREEN VEGETABLES WITH A HOT NUT CRUST

Preparation time: 15 minutes
Cooking time: 25–30 minutes
Serves 2

4 tablespoons walnut or sesame oil
Selection of prepared green vegetables, (about 450g/1lb total
  weight), such as broccoli florets, shredded green cabbage, chopped
  celery, chicory leaves and sliced fennel
2 tablespoons mixed nuts, such as almonds, walnuts and Brazil nuts
1–2 fresh red chillies, seeded and finely chopped
2 slices soft goat's cheese or sheep's cheese, each slice about
  1cm/½in thick
Chopped fresh coriander, to garnish

1. Preheat the oven to 220°C/fan 200°C/gas mark 7. Pour
the walnut or sesame oil into a large, non-stick roasting
tin and heat in the oven for a few minutes until hot.

2. Place the prepared mixed vegetables in the tin, turning
them in the hot oil until evenly coated all over. Roast
in the oven for about 15–20 minutes or until the
vegetables are slightly browned and crisped, stirring
once or twice during cooking.

3. Meanwhile, crush the nuts using a pestle and mortar,
or by placing them in a polythene food bag, and rolling
over them with a bottle or rolling pin. Add the chillies,
then sprinkle this mixture evenly over the vegetables
for the last few minutes of the roasting time.

4. When the vegetables are ready, remove them from the
oven and spoon onto two warmed serving plates. Roll

the cheese slices over the inside of the cooling roasting tin to coat them with any leftover nut and chilli mix. Place the cheese on top of the vegetables, then sprinkle any remaining nut mix over the top. Garnish with chopped coriander and serve on its own or with a mixed leaf salad.

This recipe is suitable for vegetarians.

HARVEST VEGETABLE CURRY

This spicy mixed root vegetable combination is slowly simmered on the hob to create a richly flavoured authentic vegetable curry.

Preparation time: 20 minutes
Cooking time: 50 minutes
Serves 2

1 tablespoon olive oil
1 small red onion, chopped
1 small fresh green or red chilli, seeded and finely chopped
1 clove garlic, crushed
1 teaspoon *each* ground coriander, ground cumin and turmeric
225g (8oz) can chopped tomatoes
200ml (7fl oz) vegetable stock
450g (1lb) mixed root vegetables (prepared weight), such as sweet
  potato, carrot, parsnip, swede and celeriac, cut into small dice
Freshly ground black pepper, to taste
1–2 tablespoons chopped fresh coriander

1. Heat the olive oil in a saucepan, add the onion, chilli and garlic and sauté for about 5 minutes or until softened. Stir in the ground spices and cook gently for 1 minute, stirring.

2. Stir in the tomatoes and their juice, the stock and root vegetables and season with black pepper, mixing well. Bring to the boil, then reduce the heat, cover and simmer for about 40 minutes or until the vegetables are tender, stirring occasionally. Add a little extra hot stock if needed during cooking.

3. Stir in the chopped coriander and serve on its own or with cooked brown rice.

Cook's Tips

- The selection of vegetables you use for this curry is really up to you. Root vegetables work particularly well, but try adding other vegetables such as cauliflower florets, green beans, courgettes and so on, to ring the changes.

- If you like particularly hot curries, increase the quantities of ground spices a little to suit your taste.

This recipe is suitable for vegetarians.

ROAST VEGETABLES WITH CHÈVRE BLANC

Preparation time: 15 minutes
Cooking time: 25 minutes
Serves 2

2–3 tablespoons olive oil
Selection of prepared fresh vegetables (about 450g/1lb total weight),

such as red and green peppers, courgettes, chicory, fennel, celery, red onions and kohlrabi, cut roughly into bite-sized chunks
8–12 cloves garlic (left unpeeled), or to taste
2 slices chèvre blanc cheese, each about 2cm (3/4in) thick
Freshly ground black pepper, to taste
Cayenne pepper, to taste
Chopped fresh parsley or shredded fresh basil leaves, to garnish (optional)

1. Preheat the oven to 220°C/fan 200°C/gas mark 7. Pour the olive oil into a large, non-stick roasting tin and heat in the oven for a few minutes until hot.

2. Place the prepared mixed vegetables and garlic cloves in the tin, turning them in the hot oil until evenly coated all over. Roast in the oven for 10 minutes, then stir and roast for a further 5 minutes or so until cooked to your liking.

3. Place the cheese slices over the vegetables and roast in the oven for a further 5 minutes or so until the cheese begins to brown.

4. Spoon the roast vegetables and cheese onto two warmed serving plates or bowls. Season with a sprinkling of black pepper and cayenne pepper, garnish with chopped parsley or basil, if desired, and serve. The garlic cloves can be eaten whole or squeezed over the vegetables.

This recipe is suitable for vegetarians.

PUMPKIN OR SQUASH RISOTTO WITH PECORINO CHEESE

Preparation time: 15 minutes
Cooking time: 40–50 minutes
Serves 2

1 medium pumpkin or squash (about 675–900g/1½ –2lb
  unprepared weight)
3 tablespoons olive oil
3 shallots or 1 onion, sliced
850ml (1½ pints) hot vegetable stock
1–2 cloves garlic, finely chopped
425g (15oz) uncooked brown rice
115g (4oz) Pecorino Romano cheese, grated
Freshly ground black pepper, to taste
Chopped fresh coriander or parsley, to garnish

1. Prepare the pumpkin or squash. Cut it in half and
scoop out and discard the seeds. Scoop out most of the
flesh (leaving a little to keep the sides firm) and cut it
into small cubes. Reserve the two shells and set aside.

2. Heat the olive oil in a pan, add the shallots or onion
and sauté for about 5 minutes or until softened. Add
the chopped pumpkin or squash flesh together with
225ml (8fl oz) of the hot stock and cook for 5 minutes.

3. Add the garlic, the rest of the stock and the rice and stir
to mix. Bring to the boil, then reduce the heat and
simmer until the rice is cooked and has absorbed all the
liquid, stirring frequently. Add a little extra hot stock,
if necessary.

4. Meanwhile, place the pumpkin or squash shells in a
large separate pan of boiling water and simmer for

about 20 minutes or until the flesh inside the shells has softened. Drain, then remove the shells from the pan, dry off the outside and pour away any excess liquid from the inside. Set aside and keep warm.

5. Stir most of the cheese into the cooked risotto and season with black pepper, then pile this mixture into the prepared pumpkin or squash shells and sprinkle with the remaining grated cheese. Garnish with chopped coriander or parsley and serve.

Variation

- Use 1 red onion in place of the shallots or standard (white) onion.

This recipe is suitable for vegetarians.

DESSERTS

Some people are sweet-toothed and some savoury: if sweet is your thing then here are some delicious ideas to complete your meal. Fruit, in the main, should be eaten on an empty stomach; if left to sit on top of a full stomach it can cause acidity. Some fruit such as melons contain amino acids that trigger the stomach to release its contents into the intestine just twenty minutes after the food has been eaten. This is fine if the only thing in the stomach is melon, but if it contains other foods as well the result can be a disrupted digestion.

It is best to limit your fruit intake to breakfast and for desserts follow the fab ideas below.

Greek-style yoghurt

Preparation time: 5 minutes
Cooking time: N/A
Serves 2

Natural Greek sheep's and goat's yoghurt
Runny (clear) honey, to taste
1–2 tablespoons (shelled) pistachio nuts, finely chopped

1. Spoon some yoghurt into two serving bowls. Drizzle a little honey over each portion to taste, then sprinkle with some chopped pistachio nuts.

2. Serve as it is or lightly fold the ingredients together before serving. Serve chilled.

Variation

• Other chopped nuts such as toasted hazelnuts or pine nuts may be substituted for the pistachio nuts.

Spiced grilled fruit with honey & yoghurt

Fresh fruits are brushed with a spiced honey glaze, then lightly grilled and served warm with Greek yoghurt, to create this very tempting dessert.

Preparation time: 20 minutes
Cooking time: 10–12 minutes
Serves 2

2 tablespoons runny (clear) honey
1 tablespoon fresh unsweetened apple juice
1/2 teaspoon ground mixed spice

½ ripe mango, peeled and sliced off the stone into thick strips
½ medium fresh pineapple, peeled, cored and sliced
1 eating apple, peeled, cored and cut into wedges or thick slices
1 pear or papaya, peeled, cored (or seeded) and cut into wedges or
 thick slices
2–4 good dollops of natural Greek sheep's and goat's yoghurt

1. Preheat the grill to high. Cover the rack in a grill pan with foil and set aside. Mix the honey with the apple juice and mixed spice in a large bowl. Add the prepared mango, pineapple, apple and pear or papaya and toss to coat all over with the honey mixture.

2. Arrange the fruit in a single layer over the prepared grill rack, then drizzle any remaining honey mixture over the top. Grill the fruit for about 10–12 minutes or until slightly softened, tinged brown and hot, turning once or twice.

3. Spoon the mixed grilled fruit onto two serving plates and drizzle with any cooking juices. Spoon a dollop or two of Greek yoghurt alongside and serve immediately. Drizzle the yoghurt with a little extra honey, if desired.

Variations

• Use ground cinnamon or ginger in place of mixed spice.

• Freshly squeezed orange juice or fresh unsweetened pineapple juice may be substituted for the apple juice.

This recipe is suitable for vegetarians.

Sticky baked bananas

Peeled bananas are sliced lengthways, drizzled with a combination of orange juice, honey and ground cinnamon, then lightly oven baked, to create this tasty and warming dessert.

Preparation time: 10 minutes
Cooking time: 20 minutes
Serves 2

2 tablespoons freshly squeezed orange juice
2 tablespoons runny (clear) honey
1/2–1 teaspoon ground cinnamon, or to taste
2 firm, ripe bananas

1. Preheat the oven to 180°C/fan 160°C/gas mark 4. Put the orange juice, honey and cinnamon in a small bowl and mix well.

2. Peel the bananas and slice each one in half lengthways, then place in an ovenproof dish. Pour the orange juice mixture over the banana halves, then turn them in the mixture to coat all over.

3. Cover and bake in the oven for about 20 minutes, or until the bananas are beginning to soften. Serve the hot bananas on warmed serving plates (slice the bananas diagonally, if desired) with the sauce drizzled over.

Variations

• Ground mixed spice or ginger may be substituted for the cinnamon.

- Use fresh peaches or nectarines (peeled, stoned and sliced into wedges) in place of the bananas.

Cook's Tip

- For extra crunch and appeal, serve the baked bananas with a sprinkling of chopped nuts (such as hazelnuts or pistachios) or seeds (such as linseeds or toasted sesame seeds).

This recipe is suitable for vegetarians.

CINNAMON-SPICED APPLE WEDGES WITH HONEY

Apple wedges are lightly fried, then tossed with chopped dried apricots, a drizzle of honey and a dusting of ground cinnamon, to create this simple but delicious dessert.

Preparation time: 15 minutes
Cooking time: 15 minutes
Serves 2

3 eating apples, such as Golden Delicious or Fuji
1 tablespoon sunflower oil
55g (2oz) ready-to-eat dried apricots, finely chopped
1 tablespoon runny (clear) honey, or to taste
1/2 teaspoon ground cinnamon, or to taste

1. Peel the apples, then cut each one into quarters and remove and discard the cores and pips. Cut each apple quarter into 2–3 even wedges (each whole apple is cut into 8–12 even wedges). Place the apple wedges in a non-stick frying pan, add the sunflower oil and toss gently to mix until the apples are coated all over. Spread out the apple wedges in a single layer in the pan.

2. Heat the pan over a medium heat and cook the apple wedges for about 10 minutes or until they are beginning to lightly brown or caramelise slightly, turning the apple wedges occasionally but being careful not to break them up. Add the dried apricots, honey and cinnamon and cook for a further 2–3 minutes, or until the apples are tender, turning occasionally.

3. Serve the hot cooked apple wedges on their own or with a good dollop of natural Greek sheep's and goat's yoghurt.

Variations

- Use ground mixed spice in place of cinnamon.

- Sultanas, raisins or dried sweetened cranberries may be substituted for the apricots.

This recipe is suitable for vegetarians.

APRICOT YOGHURT ICE

This refreshing orange-scented apricot ice creates a lovely, light dessert, suitable at any time of year. It makes a great freezer-standby dessert.

Preparation time: 10 minutes, plus freezing time
Cooking time: N/A
Serves 4

55g (2oz) ready-to-eat dried apricots, roughly chopped
4 tablespoons freshly squeezed orange juice
400g (14oz) can apricots in fruit juice
250g (9oz) natural Greek sheep's and goat's yoghurt
2 tablespoons runny (clear) honey, or to taste
Small fresh mint sprigs, to decorate (optional)

1. Place the dried apricots and orange juice in a blender or food processor and blend until roughly smooth. Add the canned apricots and their juice and blend until smooth and combined. Add the yoghurt and honey and blend until well mixed. Taste the mixture and blend in a little extra honey, if desired.

2. Pour the apricot mixture into a chilled, shallow, plastic freezer-proof container and level the surface. Cover and freeze for 1 1/2–2 hours, or until mushy.

3. Spoon the mixture into a chilled bowl and mash with a fork until smooth (or leave the mixture in the container and mash it well). Return the mixture to the container and level the surface, then cover and freeze for a further 1–1 1/2 hours or until mushy. Turn the mixture into a chilled bowl once again and mash until smooth (or mash it again in the container), then return to the container as before. Cover and freeze until firm.

4. Transfer the container of frozen yoghurt ice to the fridge (or a cool room temperature) about 30 minutes before serving, to soften a little. Serve in scoops on its own or with a selection of fresh mixed berries. Decorate with mint sprigs, if desired.

This recipe is suitable for vegetarians.

ENTERTAINING ON THE DETOX PROGRAMME

Entertaining means providing your guests with pleasant surroundings, wonderful food and great company. Entertaining on the Detox Programme is all of this with the bonus of great, healthy food that will do them good. Let your guests know that you are on the programme, but only after they have eaten and told you how delicious everything was. They will be amazed that the sumptuous meal you will have been able to prepare from the recipes and food lists can be so good for you. Before you know it you will have all your friends following the programme and asking you for your advice!

As well as you telling them about the detox, they will undoubtedly tell you how good you are looking and how much the programme suits you – this is a really positive aspect of the programme and should be appreciated. You have to put a lot of work and self-control into the programme, and it is right that you should benefit from the results, both inside and out.

On the following pages are some suggested menus from the recipes given above.

Menu 1

Olives to nibble
*
Pea and onion soup
*
Smoked haddock with pine nut and coriander crumble
*
Spiced grilled fruit with honey and yogurt

Menu 2

Prawn and broccoli stir-fry
*
Chargrilled salmon with watercress
*
Apricot yogurt ice

Menu 3

Beetroot and fennel salad with mixed nuts
*
Grilled cod and colcannon
*
Sticky baked bananas

Menu 4

Crunchy red coleslaw with flaked mackerel

*

Salade niçoise

*

Selection of fresh fruit and goat's cheese

Menu 5

Selection of three-bean salad and hummus with mini rice cakes

*

Harvest vegetable curry

*

Cinammon spiced apple wedges with honey

It is likely that your guests will be drinking wine. Chilled grape juice with sparkling water, or sparkling water with a few drops of angostura bitters and a twist of lime could be your detox alternative – much more refreshing and it guarantees you a clear head in the morning.

LOGISTICAL PROBLEMS AND SOLUTIONS

No time to have a meal

There are always times during the week when you would skip a meal if you were eating normally. While you are following the Detox Programme you should never miss a meal. This doesn't mean that you must stop everything, whatever the situation, and demand to have food. But it does mean that you should always be prepared and carry some form of light snack that will tide you over until it is more convenient to eat.

Carry a larger than usual handbag or briefcase when you are detoxing and make sure that you have something for emergency measures; rice cakes, a pot of hummus or (in cooler weather only) goat's cream cheese, and a small plastic bag of dried fruit and nuts. If you prefer cheese, then a few cubes of feta in a bag will 'feed' your body. These should take up little space and will keep the hunger satisfied.

It is also worth having a little snack box with you so that you can always have a little something to eat before you go out to eat. When we are sat at the table in a restaurant, making the right detox food decisions if you are starving hungry can be difficult and it is easy to be swayed by the bread basket. If you snack before you go, it takes the edge off your hunger and then you can happily make the right choice without wanting to eat the actual menu card.

Being out with people who are not detoxing

Whatever you do, don't hide the fact that you are detoxing. Talk about the programme – people will be fascinated and ask lots of questions. This means that they will understand your situation, so any decisions about eating out or getting food will automatically include your needs. If you keep the programme quiet it will be harder to 'shoehorn' your requests into their chosen meal plans.

There will always be some people who try to make you break the programme as soon as they see the opportunity – 'just one glass of wine won't hurt, surely?' – so letting the whole group know the situation will make it easier to ignore this person.

Talking about the Detox Programme also puts it into perspective for yourself. It is likely that at times you will just be 'doing the programme' as it will have become a part of your everyday life, but it is very important to remind yourself just how effective the programme is and how great you feel. Telling people about it makes you become totally aware of everything that is happening to you and everything that you are doing for yourself.

There's only fast food available

Fast food is great! Apples, carrots, cauliflower, rice cakes and hummus are fast food, nuts and seeds are fast food – everything is a fast food if all you have to do is reach into your handbag to get it out. Don't be caught out thinking there is nothing to eat when your friends get a takeaway – have your own takeaway with you all the time.

Feeling hungry while shopping, or meeting friends for coffee

Again, if you have food with you, you are likely to be able to satisfy any hunger pangs without leaving the programme. Drinking something will also take away any immediate hunger, so stopping for a cup of herbal tea will give your feet a rest and your body some refreshment.

If you are having tea or coffee with friends, most cafés offer hot water or herbal teas as an alternative. And if your friends are having cake or biscuits you should ask if the café can supply any fresh fruit. If there is still nothing to eat, just nibble discreetly on some nuts from your bag.

Eating out and there's nothing detox on the menu

Whether in the most expensive restaurant or the cheapest you can always call the waiter or waitress over and ask if they can put together a salad or a plate of assorted vegetables. Even if a restaurant doesn't show salad anywhere on the menu they will always serve salad garnish on some of their dishes, so asking them to put this together as a main course is easy. Side orders of vegetables are normally served without dressings (check with the waiter or waitress) so these are an obvious option. You can either just order side dishes or ask for these to be made into a main course. Potatoes can be the saving vegetable. If they are baked – great. If they are roasted in vegetable or olive oil – great. And if there is nothing else you can think of then fries cooked in vegetable or seed oil are fine – unsalted!

If you need to eat carbohydrate and there are no potatoes or brown rice available then you may have a small portion of wild or white rice – the less refined the better. But this should only be in extreme cases of hunger!

Chinese or Indian restaurants are likely to cause the biggest problems as these are really the only restaurants that don't serve vegetables unless they are cooked in spicy, creamy sauces or with monosodium glutamate. If this is the case then prawns are usually on offer in some form.

Any sauce on them should be wiped off with your knife and fork, and if you eat them with plain boiled rice you will not be harming the Detox Programme. Just make sure your next meal contains lots of fresh vegetables to make up the shortfall. In Chinese restaurants you may see 'stir-fry' on the menu. Ask if this is without sauce and simply tossed in spices and oil – if so, tuck in!

Restaurants are much more user-friendly than they used to be, and many pride themselves on being able to provide almost anything that you request – put them to the test!

PART 3

Maintenance and Enhancement

6

Diary of a Detox

The easiest way to demonstrate life on the Detox Programme is to take you through the day-to-day diary of someone who has actually done it. This chapter will take you through six days of the programme: two from the start, two from the middle and two towards the end. It shows the different stages you will go through, what to expect to feel and what might happen over the 30 days.

The person who wrote this diary was single, living with a partner and working. As far as the Detox Programme is concerned, being single or married makes no difference. You will either be coaxing your partner to eat the same food or cooking for one – simply adapt the quantities to suit.

Working at home, working at the office, not working or being a mother/father with children at home and so on, are surprisingly interchangeable situations. The adaptations you have to make due to being at work or in a meeting are the same as those you have to make at home surrounded by young children – these are all distractions, and the diary simply demonstrates that, with a little preparation and planning, you can adapt the programme to suit any lifestyle.

Eating out or entertaining hold the same opportunities and problems for everyone. You will see that all these demands can be easily coped with while you are on the programme.

DAY 1, SUNDAY

Try to be busy on the first day – make sure you have all the right food available and then get going.

The temptation to spend the day with the sole focus of FOOD will be exhausting and very negative.

Got up and took a shower as usual and then turned the shower to cold for approximately five seconds, legs only – that will do for Day 1, I think. After drying off I tried out the dry-skin brushing, then realised I should have done it before my shower but all the same, felt very warm and my skin was buzzing – felt like I had done a reasonable amount of exercise already.

I decided to clear out the cellar. *After a breakfast of hot water with lemon juice, pears, sheep's yogurt, sunflower seeds sprinkled on top and some grated ginger*, I set to work.

I also decided to start gently. The 47 trips up the stairs out into the garden carrying large boxes of rubbish would count as my 20 minutes of exercise for the day – it took two hours. I drank about four cups of hot water and found that it actually had quite a lot of flavour.

Lunch was a baked potato, the flesh mixed up with one teaspoon of olive oil to make it creamy and feta cheese melted on top. All this was served with grated beetroot on top – strangely and surprisingly delicious.

I finished my lunch and set about finally sorting out

my holiday photos, something I have been needing to do for a long time. Several trips to the toilet later – just proves that my body is not used to having so much fluid to deal with – I start to feel like I am actually beginning to flush out. I didn't feel tired or lethargic at any stage during the day and actually feel as if I have got more done than I ever do on a normal Sunday. Perhaps it is symbolic that I chose to 'clean out' and 'sort out' my life on the day that I start to 'clean out' and 'sort out' my body.

Supper at 6.45 of roast vegetables: leeks, onions, fennel, courgettes and broccoli with creamy goat's cheese melted on top and served on a bed of short grain brown rice. I felt like I needed a dessert but ended up with a handful of almonds which had more flavour than I previously remember them having, not as good as sticky toffee pudding but I suppose sacrifice is the name of the game . . .

When it came to bedtime I still felt quite alert so I massaged both my legs and arms with my normal moisturiser and went to bed.

Had a really good night's sleep.

DAY 2, MONDAY

Woke up really invigorated this morning, could be just in my mind so we shall see – didn't want to get out of bed but didn't feel as if I needed more sleep. Went to the gym for half an hour and did ten minutes each on the treadmill, step machine and bike.

Got home, showered and then splashed about in the bath in cold water. Definitely prefer just turning the shower to cold for a few minutes as running the bath was time-consuming. Drank the hot water and dry-skin brushed – fitting it all in is OK but will require concentration – and yes, I should have brushed *before*. Note to self . . .

Had the same as yesterday for breakfast. Thought that I was being bad not to use my imagination with all the new fruit to try, but then realised that I have had toast and coffee every morning for the last 22 years so having the same while on the detox should be no problem.

Had a busy morning in the office and every time I came to drink my hot water it was cold water – just as refreshing. My skin seems to be a tad greasy today. We had a conversation across the office about skin care and no one asked me what I did to keep looking young and beautiful – I suspect it was a tactful way of saying I didn't! I am surprised this has happened so quickly but it is only to be expected if I am cleansing myself.

Lunch was last night's leftover roast vegetables, adding a little quinoa for bulk and then I panicked that I would get hungry so ordered a salad from the corner sandwich bar. I probably overdid the salad. I asked for a large green salad and couldn't actually finish it off.

Developed a very mild headache this afternoon so I drank some camomile tea and did some deep breathing. Feels better but not completely gone. This might last a while so I will take a rest as soon as possible, but in the meantime it's meetings, meetings, meetings.

Needed to drive into town, normally I load up for the two-hour drive with snacks and potato crisps, but had *water and a bag of almonds to nibble on* – felt very virtuous but most of them are now in the well of my car. Drank quite a lot of water but realised that there was nowhere to stop to visit the toilet on the journey so stopped drinking quite as much.

I met up with an old schoolfriend for supper and called ahead to warn her that I was 'detoxing' and would bring my own food if necessary but the menu was: *olives to start as appetisers, black and green. Steamed vegetables: carrot, cauliflower, white and red cabbage all mixed with brown rice and sesame and cumin seeds. She had yogurt and straw-berries for dessert and I just had the strawberries – it couldn't have been more detox if she had tried.*

Drove home feeling tired but happy that I had managed to eat out without breaking the programme or disrupting my host's evening. Went to bed with the headache, still mild, but not unmanageable – proof that my body is beginning its clean out. Must remember to vacuum the car ... or get a bib.

DAY 14, FRIDAY

I am working in town today and so staying with a friend. Got up feeling really good. Before I 'showered and brushed' or should I say 'brushed and showered' – finally got it the right way round – I weighed myself. I have been tempted to do this every day since I started but decided that I would only weigh in twice – in the middle and at the end. I know the programme is not about weight loss, but as I am doing all this exercise and feel so good and 'lean and clean' it would be the icing on the cake.

I have lost 5lb – feel sooo virtuous. This is good because it is not too much for two weeks but also accounts for any actual gain of weight due to fat converting to toned muscle. This makes me feel even better and so I treat myself for breakfast by having something different from my usual pears and yogurt topped with seeds – *I mix together grapes, apples and strawberries and stir in some freshly grated root ginger. Steady, I may be enjoying it.*

I have begun to see my plate as 'energy food' and have become a bit obsessive about my superfoods. If they are as good as they are supposed to be I'm going to be super-woman before you know it.

Went to work and had a massage treatment at lunchtime – that was wonderful, but I wish I had booked it for this evening as I really felt like making the most of feeling relaxed. But I had to go straight back to work and then drive home afterwards.

Usually I feel tired driving home this late in the week, but my massage must have been more invigorating than I thought. Came home via the gym and someone said that my skin was positively glowing – and they didn't even know I was on the Detox Programme. It must look as good as it feels.

Supper was delicious. I was cooking for two – and number two had made it quite clear that he was not on the detox! Grilled salmon fillets on a bed of watercress, lightly stir-fried red cabbage and red onions and chargrilled courgettes, all drizzled with olive oil and lime juice and a handful of black olives. We finished with a winter-fruits frozen yogurt (sheep's).

The only thing I crave is a glass of cool white wine, but *apple juice and fizzy water makes a suitable alternative ... who am I trying to kid?!*

Before going to bed, which is getting later and later as I get more and more energy – it must be difficult to live with a 'detoxer' as you can see their boundless energy while you still feel exhausted at the end of every day – I smooth in some detox massage oil. May as well keep everything working on my behalf while I am snoozing.

DAY 15, SATURDAY

Got up quite early today as we have friends coming to stay and I need to make the house look less like a war zone and then get some shopping done. I wonder if they will notice, unprompted, that I have shed a few pounds and look a little more lively than I normally do. Hot lemon water while sitting up in bed looking at the post, skin brush and then a quick shower. *Breakfast consisted of a pear and a handful of nuts and seeds in the car on the way to the supermarket.*

Not much lunch to speak of as we walk our friends around town and take them for afternoon tea. *I have herbal tea and a fresh fruit salad from the coffee shop and a slightly mangled banana from the depths of my handbag, taking my life in my hands* while they have coffee and cake. Normally I would find this hard to deal with, but the idea of caffeine seems to fill me with horror and the cake would feel far too stodgy.

We are eating out this evening and I am interested to know how easy it is to do this as, so far, I have managed to avoid it.

The restaurant came out on top. I had mixed olives to start – the selection of breads with olive oil that the others had did look rather good, but again I didn't miss the bread as I feel it would mess up my clean insides – and I had taken the precaution and waded my way through a pot of my delicious home-made roast veg paste (whiz up all leftover roast veg with a few tomatoes and store in an airtight container) with some celery to take the edge of my hunger. Anyway, I digress, roast monkfish on a bed of roast peppers with a hazelnut oil and lime dressing, all with a side salad of rocket and pecorino romano shavings in olive oil and lemon – it actually looked much nicer than the risotto that the others chose so I was happily full and satisfied, without feeling bloated.

I feel really self-righteous at the moment but am keeping it to myself – we had an in-depth discussion over dinner about what food was good and why I couldn't eat certain things. At the end of the day I think if we went back to an original diet; that is, nothing mixed – which means basically veg, fruit, nuts, beans, pulses, fish, white meat and non-dairy – then I reckon we would all be a lot cleaner and healthier.

I don't feel hungry and I'm looking forward to my weigh-in next Sunday. If I have lost even one more pound that will be absolutely superb!

I didn't massage this evening or this morning as I have awarded myself the day off for doing so well – and we gossiped late into the evening, some of us slurring a little more than is attractive!

DAY 28, WEDNESDAY

Had to get into town early to pick up some printing I have had done, so decided that a trip to the grocers was in order.

Their ready-prepared green salad looked good and so

did their giant raisins and apricots. Got a bag of mixed washed vegetables and toddled on back home.

I now feel that the programme is an integral part of my life, it's day 28 and technically I should be buying 'normal food' to celebrate completion, but that doesn't feel the right way to go about it, undoing all the good work I've put in overnight. The fact that I haven't even mentioned the self-massage and skin brushing, and so on, this morning means that I am managing to fit them in without even blinking. I have missed them out on a couple of mornings, but when I realised I definitely wished I had remembered.

Breakfast was two apples, hundreds of grapes and a handful of jumbo raisins and sultanas while I sat at my desk working – definitely could have been vastly improved with a big dollop of goat's yogurt.

Worked all morning and couldn't believe it when lunchtime arrived. *Lunch was a baked potato, green salad and a large scoop of home-made hummus – this makes the potato really creamy and actually quite wonderful.*

Still at my desk at 6.30, so nipped to the corner shop for *a tin of tuna in veg oil, and had that with the mixed vegetables and some beetroot and feta. I felt full but not over-full, and I think my tastebuds have been reborn – the flavours are quite brilliant even with something so plain.*

Loads of hot water this evening and I suspect I will have to get up in the night as a result.

Bed and 'drainage massage' before sleep. I have also noted that my sleep is very, very much deeper than it has been in ages. I honestly believe that I now go to sleep and don't wake until the alarm goes off – normally I wake a few times when turning over. This is excellent, and I hope it is one of the lasting results of detox, and I feel sure sleep makes me beautiful!

DAY 29, THURSDAY

Knew I was going to be very busy today so I started by saying my affirmations to myself several times while breathing deeply and slowly before getting out of bed:

> I am successful.
> I am healthy.
> I feel full of energy.
> I am prepared for anything.
> I've blinking done the whole programme
>   and I've reached day 29 yeeeeah!

(The last one was one of my own personalised affirmations, not in the book.) I have found that saying these makes an immediate difference, and nothing can get me down during the day because 'I am prepared for anything – bring it on.'

I did my normal morning routine and decided that I will definitely continue to turn the shower to cold but will probably only dry-skin brush every few days – wonder how long it will last.

Breakfast has settled down to yogurt, apples and grapes and I nibble on the seeds throughout the morning in the office. I put a bag of nuts and seeds in my desk at the start of the week and then I can forget having to prepare them every day.

I got out of a meeting very late and all there was to

drink was fizzy water so I feel a bit bloated – I definitely find flat or hot water easier to digest.

I didn't have time to exercise at the gym today, so I ran up and down the office stairs four times and walked around the block briskly before I drove home. I miss exercise if I don't get the chance to do at least 20 minutes a day – I generally do 40 minutes, which is more than required but feels fine.

I still think I can feel the benefit from my detox body massage on Saturday – I was a bit drowsy immediately afterwards but seem to have even more energy now. My skin feels wonderful – ten years younger without the surgery.

I'm afraid I didn't get time for lunch so I had the last of my rice cakes with some feta cheese at my desk – the feta tastes very salty now, so my tastebuds must be completely clean and detecting every flavour I subject them to.

Tomorrow is the last day of the Detox Programme for me. I actually think I will miss a lot of the programme, and will probably keep to it during the week and then gradually phase in the things I have missed at weekends. The idea of eating bread or meat isn't very appealing. I will have a glass of wine, but that will be the only thing that I think I have really missed.

As I am working tomorrow evening – my 'last evening' – we planned to eat out tonight to 'celebrate' my achievement: *red mullet and salmon on a green bean and onion salad, dressed in oil and vinegar, followed by grilled goat's cheese roulade on a bed of roast vegetables and hazelnuts, all washed down with mineral water* – well done me!

Obviously your own days will be very different, but the essence of the eating and detox activities and how you fit them into your day will remain the same. There will be some days on which you do more towards the Detox Programme than on others, but you should definitely include the daily food and activity checklist items as and when required. Missing something out will not mean you should start all over again. It simply means that you will not be getting the greatest benefit from the programme – and as you can see, it really is quite easy to follow.

7

Maintaining the Detox

There are ways to 'come off' the Detox Programme, ways to prolong and maintain the programme, ways to do a 'short detox' programme and mini-fasts. All these, in combination with the full 30-day programme, will maintain a permanent state of detox for your body.

The first time you follow the programme will always be the most challenging, for you will be detoxing all the eating habits of your life to that day – 20, 30, 40 years or whatever. The second time you undertake the programme your body will remember pretty quickly how it feels to be eating well, and, as you probably have not gone back to all of your old ways anyway, your second detox will be much easier because you have done it before. Your body will respond much more immediately and the highs of energy that, on the first occasion, took between seven and 14 days to experience will be felt by the end of Week 1. However, it is still very important to detox for as long as you can, a minimum of ten days, in order to get the most benefit.

'COMING OFF' THE DETOX PROGRAMME

What you do immediately after your first Detox Programme can increase and prolong the effect of the detox by many months. But whatever you do after the programme is completed you cannot reverse the good work you have done. Even if you decide to return to burgers and caffeine you will still enjoy the benefits of detox and your body will still thank you for the 'rest and recuperation' you gave it.

On Day 30 of the programme you will be looking forward to taking yourself out to dinner or making a meal to reward yourself for all the hard work and self-control you have exercised in the previous month. You should definitely do something to mark your success, but be aware that coming off the programme is as crucial as starting it.

Over the last 30 days your body has become used to being nourished with simple foods that it can readily digest and absorb. It has become used to high nutrition. It has become used to not having to compromise or compensate for what you feed yourself, but to enjoy and benefit from everything you have done. Processed foods, preservatives, additives, chemicals and refined foods have not been part of your diet for a whole month. If you add all these foods back overnight, your body may find it difficult to digest them. This can cause constipation, indigestion, headaches, bloating, sugar highs and lows and, potentially, mood swings. If you now wish to include some or all of these 'old' foods in your diet, do so slowly and over a period of time to avoid any of these side effects. But, more importantly, if you introduce them one at a time you will be able to tell what each specific effect on you is: being tired, grouchy, having headaches or feelings of being bloated could be just a few tell-tale signs that they are not too good for you. Start to listen to your body: how is it responding? How do they make you feel?

As you start to approach Day 30 you should assess how you feel and think about the things that you wish to re-introduce once the programme has been completed. Make a list of these foods, and also note those that you have really missed. Normally, the things that you have missed will be the types of food to which you may have developed an intolerance to before going on the programme. Common examples are white bread, cheese, coffee, wine, sweet cakes, biscuits and red meat.

You should then start to think about how you will *gradually* introduce these into your programme. As I mentioned earlier, if you add them one at a time you will be able to monitor how your body responds to them. Then, if there is an adverse reaction you can exclude them or introduce them in much smaller amounts over a longer period of time.

If, for instance, you want to reintroduce bread or refined flour, don't have toast for breakfast, a sandwich for lunch and pasta for supper. It is likely that this kind of overload will make you feel bloated and sluggish. Instead you should have toast on the first day, a salad sandwich on the second and pasta for supper on the third. Check how you feel, and then increase the frequency if all seems well.

Also, make the foods you reintroduce the healthiest version available. For example, the pasta needs to be wholewheat or spelt and the bread should be wholegrain, wholemeal or pumpernickel and so on. These are not only better for you as they are more nutritious, but they are also less refined and therefore have slower-release sugars, so you shouldn't feel hungry or sluggish afterwards. If you are a chocolate lover, then keep the level of chocolate you snack on to a minimum of 60 per cent cocoa solids, organic and with fruit: you would be surprised how delicious and healthy chocolate can be – in small amounts. As I write this, there is a bag of almonds and a bar of 'smooth and rich dark chocolate (70 per cent) with raspberries' on my desk – recommended to me by my massage therapist, Debbie Hope, and very good it is too. Of course it is all in the name of research but, joking aside, it is better to be eating this than a bar of 20 per cent cocoa chocolate full of E numbers and sugar.

You may find that a slice of breakfast toast is enough to satisfy your bread requirements, so try to remember how much good you have done to your body and how reducing the amount of items such as refined flours will prolong the effects of the detox.

It is also likely that rich or very creamy foods will upset your stomach. Treat these with care. Again, excluding these foods or eating them only very occasionally will prolong the effects of your detox, and they are not nutritionally fabulous anyway.

Don't be surprised if there are some foods that you would have previously considered as regular staples in your diet but which you now find difficult to eat. Your tastes may well have changed and their flavours are no longer acceptable. These foods are generally meat and dairy foods and those with strong or salty flavours. Over a period of time you will regain your taste for them if you eat them in small amounts. But again this may be a great opportunity to cut these foods out permanently, especially if they are processed or contain a lot of additives.

MAINTAINING THE DETOX PROGRAMME

As well as watching the sorts of foods you reintroduce when you have completed the 30 days, you should also note the foods from the Detox Programme that you want to keep as a staple part of your new healthier diet. If you wish to 'stop' the programme and return to how you were eating previously, there are still parts of the programme that you can continue with without restricting your choices. Combining your eating habits in this way will supplement any areas of deficiency. Even just by keeping the superfoods as a regular part of your daily intake you will greatly improve your nutrition levels as well as maintaining your detox.

The easiest parts of the programme to stick with when you have finished are those that take very little time and can be done without really having to think about them, the things that have become a habit. Remember, good habits are brilliant, as they require no effort – they are habits.

Drink a cup of hot water and lemon juice first thing every morning

Whether you are on the programme or not, starting the day with hot water and lemon is very refreshing, cleansing for your liver and invigorating. It is just as easy to add lemon juice as it is to put a teaspoon of coffee or a teabag in your mug – and much better for you. A few squirts of lemon juice with water 30 minutes before you eat will also take the edge of your appetite and help you make good food choices instead of just grabbing anything because you are feeling incredibly hungry.

During the day drink 1.5 litres (2³/₄ pints) of water

Once you have got into the habit of drinking lots of water during the programme it is much easier to carry on than to stop. Your body will have become used to the extra fluids, and reducing the amount will make you thirsty. There is no good reason to stop the water intake – so don't!

Keep up with the superfoods

We all have standard foods that we always 'have in'; the types of food that we know we can use to whip up a feast from just a few staple ingredients if anyone descends on us unannounced or if we just get hungry. We have favourite quick recipes and we have what I call fridge food – foods that you open the fridge door, reach in for, and start munching there and then.

Well, if you can make your staples consist of foods from the superfood list, your quick-fix lunches or suppers consist mostly of superfoods, and if you can find a fridge snack that is only superfood, then you are on to a winning formula – quick, tasty, nutritious no-brainers. Brilliant.

Eat three meals every day, or three to five smaller meals

Three meals a day is very important, even if they are non-detox meals. Leaving long gaps in between meals or skipping meals will disrupt the body's delicate metabolism and push it into starvation mode. Eating three to five smaller meals a day is infinitely preferable to having two or three meals with large gaps in between.

The effects

Continuing with the aspects of the programme listed above will:

- Act as a tonic to your liver and kidneys.

- Cleanse your palate and intestines.

- Flush out any toxins you consume.

- Keep the pH balance in your body regulated.

- Maintain a good metabolic rate.

- Keep energy levels constant and ensure mood swings are less frequent.

Coupled with your new detoxed body, these habits will maintain a constant cleansing process. They should take no more than five minutes out of your day.

FASTING, MINI-FASTS AND MINI-MINI- FASTS

I have never been into fasting. I like my food too much and believe that fuelling my body with optimum nutrition is a better way to support and cleanse myself than not feeding my body anything for a period of time. However, I am open-minded and I know that for some people, the idea of fasting is a good one, as they feel that they are really having a thorough cleanse.

Fasting has been popular for many hundreds of years and there are claims that it is a way of totally cleansing your insides. It means eating nothing and drinking only water. Fasting allows the body to cleanse itself of waste and empty the systems of all residual foods. Once clear of waste, the body can absorb and use all nutritional foods more efficiently. It also facilitates the release of hormones that stimulate the immune system.

Various different lengths of fast can be undertaken, but if you wish to complete a fast of three days or more it must always be under the supervision of your doctor. The side effects of long-term fasting – without correct supervision and instruction – can do more harm than good. Literally starving your body for more than 24 hours will lead to feelings of weakness, nausea and dizziness, muscle fatigue and dehydration. If you try to operate normally – going to work, looking after the family and so on – you are likely to suffer major lapses in concentration and extreme fatigue. Any existing health conditions will be exacerbated by lack of nourishment.

There are other forms of fasting that are less severe and,

in my view, much more effective. Restricting your diet to certain types of cleansing foods for between 24 and 48 hours, but no longer, can help to maintain and/or boost the Detox Programme.

Once you have completed the programme you may find times when you think you have eaten too many processed foods, or have had to eat out a lot and don't feel as if you have been very kind to your body. At times like these you can try a mini-fast. You can also think about trying a mini-mini-fast more regularly – perhaps once a week on an evening when you are not going out.

If you fast after you have detoxed it will bring positive results immediately. Each time you fast you are giving your body time out; time to rest and recuperate after the many years of hard work spent digesting the 'not very nutritional' foods you have been enjoying. Fasting regularly after detox will maintain the detox at its fullest potential.

Don't just decide to fast and then starve yourself for the next few days. Fasting must be thought through, and preparation is essential if you are to get the best results.

How to fast

Check that you fulfil the necessary health requirements, as with the Detox Programme:

- You are not pregnant.

- You are not breastfeeding.

- You do not suffer from any illness or heart condition.

- You are not diabetic.

- You are not taking prescribed or recreational drugs.

- You have no doubts about your own personal health.

Decide when you want to fast and for how long – a mini-fast is 18 hours and a mini-mini-fast 14 hours.

As with the detox programme, you must start and finish gradually. Leading up to the fast you should cut out caffeine, red meat, processed foods and alcohol. The last three meals before your fast should all be from the Detox Programme.

Throughout the fast you should:

- Drink plenty of hot water, lemon juice and honey.

- Take vitamin C supplements every four hours.

- Drink at least 2 litres (3¹/₂ pints) of fluid in the form of water, herbal teas, or apple, grape or lemon juice over the period of the day. The amount is more than the normal detox as you will not be getting any fluids from foods.

- Have some black grapes to nibble on in case your hunger becomes unbearable.

Once you have finished your fast you should eat only foods from the Detox Programme for a day, and then slowly introduce normal foods in the same way you would when finishing the programme.

The mini-fast

This fast can be undertaken once a month and will give your body the 'time out' it needs to cleanse internally.

The mini-fast takes place overnight, so you are only aware of fasting for around ten waking hours, as you sleep through most of it! It lasts from 6.00 p.m. until 3.00 p.m. the following day. Having eaten detox foods during the day you should:

- At 6.00 p.m. eat a light vegetarian meal, ideally from the Detox Programme.

- Eat nothing until 3.00 p.m. the following day, but make sure you drink plenty of herbal teas, juices or water during the early evening and following day.

- At 3.00 p.m. have a light snack of fruit, salad and brown rice.

- At 6.00 p.m. have another meal of fresh fruit and vegetables.

The mini-mini-fast

This fast should be undertaken once a week and can probably be done without really noticing you are on a fast! As with the mini-fast, you are actually asleep for most of the time so it feels like a short four- or five-hour fast. But even fasting for such a short time gives your body time to process and cleanse itself.

Getting into the habit of eating your final meal of the day as early as possible will give your body a better chance to digest the foods correctly. Detox or not, the benefits of proper digestion should not be underestimated. The mini-mini-fast takes place from 6.00 p.m. to 8.00 a.m. the following day. Having eaten detox foods during the day you should:

- At 6.00 p.m. eat a light vegetarian meal, ideally from the Detox Programme.

- Eat nothing until 8.00 a.m. the following day, but make sure you drink plenty of herbal teas, juices or water during the early evening.

- At 8.00 a.m. have a light breakfast of hot water and lemon juice, fruit, goat's or sheep's yogurt and seeds.

- At lunchtime have another meal of fresh fruit and vegetables.

You have now completed a fully functional fast with all the benefits and few 'hunger pains'. NB: This fast is most effective if you have already completed the 30-day detox.

8

Second Time Around: the Short Detox

The Detox Programme is spread over 30 days to ensure that your body has time to adapt and then become used to a new, more healthy way of operating. The gradual changes become permanent if you take them slowly. It is said that if you want to give something up you should exclude it from your diet for between one and three months, after which you stop craving it. In the same way, if you want to get out of a habit, not doing it for 21 days is the time required to break it. The flip side of this is that if you want to develop a good habit or 'get into the habit' of doing something, then doing it regularly for 21 days will make it part of your normal routine.

However, there may be times when you want to follow the Detox Programme but you don't have 30 days available, or you have already completed the full programme and would like to do a shortened version once in a while. This is where the Short Detox Programme can be followed. It is slightly more severe, but as you are trying to pack 30 days into ten, then more immediate changes are required. The ten-day programme is ideally suited to those who have already completed the full programme. Indeed, you are not recommended to follow the short programme unless you have completed the full one, or it could be too much of a short, sharp, shock for your body.

If you follow the ten-day plan you will find that the reactions you got in the 30-day programme are exaggerated: headaches may be stronger but shorter-lived, tiredness will be more immediate but will last for a shorter time, energy levels will hit a high very quickly, and your skin will look dull for a couple of days and then become radiant. The ten-day detox is a complete blitz on your body, and if you are prepared for some quite remarkable changes very rapidly, it is a great experience.

All the principles and allowable foods are the same as in the 30-day programme. The difference is simply the period of time and the way you schedule and prepare your food. The differences from the 30-day programme are shown in italics.

When you start the detox programme, from Day 1 to Day 10 you must:

- Dry-skin brush every morning *and every evening*.

- Have a full-body cold shower every morning (no time to take it step by step).

- Self-massage every morning *and every evening*.

- Drink a cup of hot water, *honey* and lemon juice first thing every morning.

- During the day drink 2 litres (3½ pints) of water.

- Have superfoods make up part of every meal (yes, every meal).

- Take multivitamin supplements *every day*.

- Eat a minimum of three meals every day.

- Have short grain brown rice, once a day, every day.

- Have three portions of *raw vegetables every day.*

- Have three portions of fruit every day. NB: *You must not eat fruit for any meal other than breakfast.*

- Have a selection of salad, non-dairy yogurt or cheese, pulses, nuts and herbs every day.

- *Take 40 minutes' exercise every day.*

- *Have 15 minutes' relaxation every day.*

- *Have ten minutes of quality breathing every day.*

- Say five affirmations and have five visualisations ten times each day.

- Smile or laugh heartily every day.

- *Exfoliate every other day.*

- Use a detox blend of oils on your body or add to the bath or shower every day.

- Have four treatments during the ten days; these can be any detoxifying treatment: body wraps, aromatherapy, reflexology, facials, and so on.

DRY-SKIN BRUSHING

1. Find a natural-bristle brush or loofah, or a dry flannel or mitt. Whichever you use should be firm but not hard, since you will be brushing your skin quite vigorously all over your body. The skin on your stomach is softer than on your shins or forearms. Do not wet or moisturise the skin, as this may cause dragging.

2. Undress to your underwear or, preferably, take all your clothes off. Stand or sit in a position that gives you access to all parts of your body – the edge of the bed with your feet on pillows is quite good, or else try sitting on the edge of the bath with one foot up on the toilet seat if it is close enough.

3. Start at the feet and systematically work up towards the top of your body. All strokes should be towards the heart – the heart is a wonderful machine for pumping blood down and throughout the body, but both blood and lymph need extra help to work against gravity to return through the system. If you brush away from the heart it may cause faintness or disrupt the normal flow. Each stroke should be long and firm. Place the brush or mitt on your ankle and firmly brush up to your knee. Repeat until you have covered the entire calf and shin several times. When you have completed the lower leg, move up to your knee. The next strokes should run from your knee to the top of your thigh and over your buttocks.

4. Then brush both arms, from the wrist to the shoulder. The neck and shoulder area should be treated more gently as the flesh here is very delicate. Work from the top of your arm, up and over your shoulder, and gently up your neck to the base of your skull.

5. When brushing your stomach, use gentle, circular strokes in a clockwise direction. This will follow the flow in your intestines and not disrupt any bowel functions.

6. You must only brush your face with a soft facial brush or flannel, as the skin here is very delicate and can be damaged if the brush is too hard.

The whole process should only take three or four minutes, and you should feel invigorated when you have finished. Your skin will tingle and you should feel quite warm, as you will have stimulated and increased your circulation. After a few sessions you will soon notice a difference in your skin: it feels smoother, with a softer texture, and the dry patches will all have disappeared. Just spend a little time each day and you will be pleasantly surprised.

COLD SHOWER EVERY MORNING

If you are doing the ten-day programme, then it's no more Mr Nice Guy. When you have finished bathing or showering in the mornings, simply turn the shower to cold, just before you are ready to finish, and let the water run over your entire body for a count of ten – counting slowly! Better still, do one whole minute. Alternatively, when you have finished your bath you can turn on the cold tap as the bathwater is draining away, cup your hands under the water and splash it all over your body.

SELF-MASSAGE

Most normal massage strokes can be converted to be used for self-massage. As long as you observe the general rules of massage, even 'made up' strokes will be perfectly acceptable and effective.

- As with dry-skin brushing, all massage strokes should be towards the heart. Pushing the blood around the system should be done in conjunction with the circulation and not against it.

- All strokes should be using either the flat hand (fingers together, palms down) or the ends of the fingers (bunched together, no fingernails).

- All massage strokes should start lightly and slowly build to a firmer, more rapid pace.

- Your flesh should be warm and relaxed before any deeper strokes can be used. Working deeply on cold, tense flesh will feel unpleasant and cause bruising.

- Massage should never be painful or sore, but massage that is too light is little better than a comforting stroke.

- You should be relaxed when carrying out self-massage, as you need to work in some awkward positions and don't want to cause any twists or injuries.

Where possible, you should make sure the room you are in is warm and quiet, perhaps with some relaxing or calming music. If the room is cold it is likely that you are not totally relaxed, which will not result in the best massage.

Use a detox massage oil, favourite cream or body lotion and apply just enough to let your hands work over the flesh firmly. If you use too much you will just slip over the skin, and if you use too little you may pull or 'burn' the skin. Reapply as necessary, and if you apply too much just wipe the excess onto another part of your body until you need it later.

Hot Lemon and Honey Water

The biggest organ of detox is the liver, so starting the day with a squeeze of fresh lemon juice in a cup of hot water will not only refresh and revitalise you but will also clean your palate and 'jump-start' your liver. Cider vinegar can be substituted, but may be a little sharp for most palates. Adding honey makes the drink even more cleansing for the bowel.

Water

You must drink 2 litres (3½ pints) of water every day. Around 80 per cent of our bodies consist of water and we need to drink to keep that level stable. In hot weather or when you are taking exercise you should increase this amount to cover the deficit. Water replenishes, cleanses, rejuvenates and restores, and is probably the most important single item in the Detox Programme.

Superfoods

You must make sure that a good selection of the following foods feature in every meal, every day. Any of the foods below can be taken in any form: raw or cooked, as a juice or tea, in a supplement (but fresh is best), as a snack or as part of a main meal:

Garlic boosts your immune system, improves circulation, reduces cholesterol, good liver tonic, reduces high blood pressure.

Grapes Powerful antioxidant, protects the heart and is good for circulation, high in water and fibre, good liver tonic.

Onions stabilise blood sugar levels, help reduce risk of heart disease, relieve congestions in airways, boost immunity.

Beetroot Cleansing and detoxifying, good for circulation, boosts immune system, strengthens blood by building up red blood cells, fights infection, energises and balances through its iron and natural sugar content, reduces inflammation.

Carrots lower blood cholesterol, increase levels of beta-carotene in the body, boost immune system, help to heal ulcers, good for teeth, hair and bones, improve condition of skin and reduce wrinkles, good liver tonic, promote general all-round health, good for the blood, heart and circulation, good for the eyes – and of course, we all know they 'help you see in the dark'!

Fennel aids digestion, eases intestinal cramps, regulates hormone levels, eases fluid retention and flatulence, helps regulate high blood pressure due to its high potassium levels.

Manuka (or organic) honey fights bacteria, provides natural energy, softening for the skin if applied topically, protects the immune system, soothes throat problems, coughs, colds and respiratory infections, relieves stomach upset.

Blueberries improve circulation, boost immune system, good antioxidant, anti-inflammatory.

Broccoli lowers risk of heart disease, lowers risk of cataracts, combats anaemia, high in nutrients and anti-oxidants, good for the digestive system and liver, mood enhancer, good for skin, contains high concentrations of folic acid for strengthening nervous system and blood. Broccoli is one of the all-round superfoods; get a taste for it now, raw dipped in hummus is delicious and unbelievably good for you.

Spinach Antioxidant, lowers risk of heart disease, may aid in reduction of progression of age-related macular degeneration, high in folates, good source of iron, relieves anaemia, high in potassium which regulates blood pressure. (Eat two or three times a week, not every day.)

Tomatoes Strong antioxidant, due to levels of lycopene, can help to prevent many illnesses from heart conditions to skin cancers, thin the blood, improve digestion, strengthen immunity, reduce liver inflammation, reported to reduce the risk of prostate cancer. Another good all-rounder, fabulous with a delicious salad dressing and one of the few foods that doesn't seem to lose any of its potency through cooking, tinned tomatoes are as good for you as raw.

Watercress boosts the immune system, protects against heart illness, good for teeth, skin, bones, muscles, heart and nervous system, good energy booster.

Cabbage (including red) Strong antioxidant, can reduce risk of cancers, good for the heart, improves digestion and digestive health, fights bacteria, tones liver, boosts immunity

SUPPLEMENTS

You must have a multivitamin supplement each day. This will ensure that any problems in the early stages of the programme will not leave your body short of essential nutrients. You must take a multivitamin every day of the intensive ten-day detox to help keep any nasty, nutritional shortfalls at bay.

THREE MEALS A DAY

You must have at least three meals per day. Breakfast should be before 9.00 a.m., lunch before 2.00 p.m. and your evening meal before 7.00 p.m. Even better is to have four to six smaller meals, which avoids large spans of time without eating and thus enables your body to fortify and detox itself without any blood-sugar lows.

BROWN RICE

You must have a large portion of brown rice every day. It acts as a sponge that travels through the gut collecting all the silt and waste, and then flushes it out. During the ten-day intensive detox you must make sure that your body is absorbing and expelling the waste as efficiently as possible.

OTHER FOOD

All the other permitted foods are fruit, raw vegetables, salads, non-dairy milk, yogurt and cheese, pulses, herbs and nuts, and are exactly the same as in the lists in Chapter 4. In order to get a healthy spread of necessary nutrients you must have some of each of these foods every day. If you miss out a food category you may begin to feel lethargic.

EXERCISE

You should do at least 40 minutes' exercise every day during the ten-day Detox Programme. Not only will this help to keep you fit and toned, but it will also ensure that your metabolic rate does not decrease or your circulation become sluggish.

BREATHING

You must have ten minutes of quality breathing every day.

1. Sit comfortably or lie down, supporting your lower back if necessary.

2. Place your hands on your stomach area with your fingertips just touching.

3. Start to breathe in through your nose very slowly to a count of four. As you inhale you should feel your stomach expand and your fingertips separate.

4. Hold your breath for four seconds and exhale slowly through your mouth to a count of eight.

5. Repeat several times as required.

It will feel strange at first as you are not used to using your muscles to expand your stomach in this way, but over a period of just a few minutes this will become more natural.

Continue this exercise for at least ten inward breaths and you should feel much more relaxed and 'centred'. Eventually you will not need to use your fingers to check that your stomach is expanding rather than your chest, and soon you will be able to carry out the exercise while you are going about your normal day-to-day business (not the lying down, but the controlled breathing!). If you ever have difficulty in dropping off to sleep, this is a far more effective way than the traditional 'counting sheep'. The chances are that you won't make it to ten, but will probably be asleep by six.

AFFIRMATIONS AND VISUALISATIONS

You must say five affirmations and do five visualisations ten times each and every day. These are ways to think and see yourself reaching your goals and achieving your own success in a personal way. When you have been doing them for a while you will notice subtle changes and your friends and colleagues will keep saying how much more positive and 'up' you seem. See pages 90 to 93 for more information on these techniques.

RELAXATION

You must have 15 minutes of total relaxation every day:

1. Find a quiet room, make sure you are warm and choose some melodic, peaceful music.

2. Lie down on the floor or sit comfortably in a chair.

3. Close your eyes and start to breathe deeply as described in the breathing exercise on page 88.

4. After breathing correctly for a couple of minutes you should find that your breathing has slowed down and it should now feel very natural.

5. When you inhale, imagine that the air you are breathing is warm and golden and is bathing your body in warm, golden, restful and positive light.

6. Now start to consider how your body is feeling. As you inhale start thinking about the feet and ankle areas of your body. Are they tense? If so, relax them.

7. As you exhale picture the air you breathe out to be the old stagnant air and the air you breathe in to be the new, fresh air.

8. Think of your calves and knees. Picture the warm air travelling through any tense muscles, bathing them in light. Exhale the stale air.

9. Picture your knee joints and your upper leg area. Breathe deeply and relax.

10. Feel the air being breathed into the groin area, relaxing the tension and soothing the pelvis. Breathe out the bad air.

11. See the golden light swirling around your stomach and abdomen, cleansing and uplifting your centre of emotion and spirit.

12. Watch the light thread its way between each rib, filling your lungs and chest cavity with warm expanding air.

13. Watch each finger fill with golden light that spreads through your fingers and lower arms.

14. Breathe in the energy into your shoulders and base of your neck. Feel your neck relax and melt into the floor or back of the chair and up into the base of your skull.

15. The light may now travel into the root of each hair follicle, making your scalp feel invigorated and tingling.

16. Each time you exhale you are breathing out waste. Each time you breathe in you are breathing in new life.

17. When you have renewed the life inside your body,

look to see where the source of your new breath and new light is coming from.

18. With your eyes still closed, look above you and see the beam of light coming down towards your body – see it feeding into your abdomen. You are connected to this light and you can take as much as you wish.

19. Breathe deeply and inhale all you need.

20. When you are ready you can start to think about bringing your consciousness back into your own body and into the room you are in.

21. Open your eyes slowly. If you are lying on the floor or bed, roll over onto your side and wait a few moments before pushing yourself up to first a sitting and then a standing position.

22. You should now feel totally relaxed and invigorated – well done!

EXFOLIATION

You must exfoliate every day. Standing on a towel, in the shower, or in the bath, take a small scoop of dry exfoliating granules and gently rub your body in firm circles, large and small, all over your body. Pay special attention to areas of hard skin such as heels, knees and elbows, and rub as hard as you find comfortable. The whole process should take about three to four minutes. As the granules fall away, either scoop them up and use again or take a new scoop. When you have completed the 'rub' you can take a long bath or shower. Then get out of the bath/shower and rub yourself dry with a towel (not one that has been rinsed in fabric conditioner, which increases its absorbency and will carry on the exfoliating process as you are drying yourself). Once dry, apply a good detox oil or cream or a good moisturiser all over your body and stay warm, perhaps by going to bed with a good book or wrapped up in front of the TV.

ADDITIONAL TREATMENTS

During the ten days you must have four detox treatments. These can be DIY or you can book yourself in with a local practitioner, salon or spa. Their treatment menus will have a long list to choose from so look for anything that is described as lymph drainage, detox, anti-cellulite, exfoliation or body wrapping. These are most likely to accelerate your detox and make you feel wonderful into the bargain. Also, any aromatherapy, massage or reflexology treatments are appropriate (see Chapter 9).

9

Ways to Enhance the Detox Programme

There are several ways in which you can enhance the Detox Programme, speed up the process, increase your awareness of your body and make the programme positively luxurious. If you choose not to do any of the treatments mentioned in this section you will not harm the detox process, but you will not be giving your body the ultimate detox environment. They are most definitely 'enhancements' and not just 'extras'. As mentioned before, detox is a combination of elements designed to provide the optimum conditions for the body to cleanse itself in every aspect: physical, emotional and mental. Any of the following treatments can also be used for stress reduction and stress management.

You have already made a decision to implement some major, exciting and positive changes in your life when you undertake the Detox Programme. So why not make it the most enjoyable experience you can by carrying out the equally beneficial but quite luxurious enhancements – you deserve them.

This would be a good time to tell you about my new range of detox products designed to accelerate your programme, to be effective and to deliver all things detox – they smell great too.

I designed them simply because there were very few products available that I thought would do the job. I also designed them so that I could supply people with everything they needed to complete their detox effectively without having to go out and about sourcing various products that would hopefully do the job. I've taken the worry out of your decision making: these do the job and are all you need – with the exception of the candle which is just a reward for you deciding to make some amazing changes in your life.

Jane Scrivner Detox products:

All instructions on how to use the products are included in the packaging.

Dry skin brush bag

Contains brushes for both body and face.

Bath and body oil

An amazing combination of nourishing jojoba and coconut oils with a deliciously effective detox blend of essential oils.

Mineral scrub

A mixture of Dead Sea salts, magnesium salts, basalt and sea salt all steeped in the detox blend of essential oils. A great dry exfoliant to slough away dead skin and leave your body warm and glowing.

Mud and quartz

This is an energising mix for the bath, or add water to form a paste to be applied to body or face for balancing nourishment. The combination of the nourishing mud and the vibrational quartz crystal will ensure that your skin, body and muscles are nourished, as well as your mind and emotions. This product recognises that sometimes your detox programme is more of a challenge for the mind than the physical body.

Candle

This three-wick candle burns for up to 40 hours, is fragranced with the Detox essential oil blend and also contains pure quartz crystals to put a positive vibe in your space and clear the room energetically.

I can recommend the whole kit to support and luxuriate your way through the programme, but if you have any alternatives that fit the descriptions included in each section then I totally encourage you to use whatever you feel appropriate. It's a great time to go through all those 'unwanted' gifts of body lotions and exfoliants and make good use of them – detox your cupboards of the tubes and bottles from your pre-detox life.

Jane Scrivner Detox treatments

Designed to work alongside the Detox Programme, these three treatments may be available in your area.

Jane Scrivner Detox total body polish

This is a total body brushing, a washing with hydromel (a mixture of honey and water), and then a full-body application of detox oils. The body is wrapped, the face massaged, and then the oils are massaged into the skin to leave you feeling cleansed and polished.

Jane Scrivner Detox Thermapeutic

This temperature technique is from Germany. It consists of wrapping the body in a cool layer, triggering the body's natural response to try to warm itself, then wrapping a tight layer of cotton and wool to trap the warmth and have the body sweat out the toxins – a kind of home sauna.

Jane Scrivner Detox Emergence

This is a reward for completing the programme: a full-body exfoliation, a full-body wrap with mud and quartz, a facial to leave the skin glowing with detox pride and then a full-body polish with oils.

Alternatively, any of the treatments described below will really help you feel good within yourself and will be good for your detox programme. Check www.janescrivner.com for practitioners in your area.

AROMATHERAPY

Many people believe that aromatherapy is simply a form of nice-smelling massage. But aromatherapy is much more than this and warrants a book of its own. However, just looking at its origins and effects will give some indication of how it can become part of your everyday life and, more specifically, part of your detox.

The plant-extracted essential oils used in aromatherapy are absorbed into our bodies via the skin or through inhalation. There used to be some doubt as to whether substances can be absorbed effectively through the skin, but this has been removed by the introduction of 'patches', for many conditions, by the pharmaceutical industry. Once in the bloodstream the molecules from the oils travel to the brain and trigger the functions appropriate to the specific oil used.

When the essential oil fragrance is inhaled through the nose, the molecules reach the brain through the thin membranes in the nasal passage and the olfactory system. Inhaling the oils is the quickest way to benefit from them (sniffing drugs has always been the quickest way to experience the effects).

The use of aromatherapy oils is recorded as early as 3000 BC. The Egyptians used oils for medical and cosmetic purposes as well as for embalming. The Greeks and Romans used them in medical practice, and medieval documents contain many references to herbal and scented oils. During the eighteenth and nineteenth centuries substances such as morphine, caffeine and quinine were recorded as ingredients obtained from medicinal plants, and even in the present day we still use plant extracts such as lavender and peppermint in common drugs. Indeed, some of the most powerful drugs available today are derived from plants: heroin, cannabis and digitalis, to name but a few.

Aromatherapy oils are, therefore, not to be regarded lightly – they can be dangerous if used incorrectly or in the wrong amounts. They are not just pleasant-smelling substances but strong, effective drugs that can have both subtle and sweeping effects on the body, mind and emotions. Many of the oils should be used only by a qualified aromatherapist, and none should be used without reference to a book or leaflet on the subject. You should not just choose an oil because you like the smell – it may have side effects that can be harmful or downright dangerous.

Essential oils should never be used if you believe you are pregnant or if you are trying to become pregnant, unless prescribed by a trained aromatherapist. Nor should essential oils ever be taken internally.

Treatment or home use

During an aromatherapy massage treatment the client lies on a massage couch, either naked or in their underwear, partially covered in towels or blankets to keep warm. The room should be warm and the practitioner should have a calm, relaxed approach. The treatment will usually last about an hour. You may feel drowsy after the session, but a glass of water will soon remedy this.

Alternatively you can use aromatherapy in your own home, as the benefit of the oils is not restricted to use in massage, and the appropriate oil can be used for almost every condition or situation. For the purpose of this book, however, I shall concentrate on those oils that are particularly useful during detox because they have cleansing and supportive properties.

Oils for detox

There are a huge number of essential oils and pre-blended mixes available today. The following list includes oils that are specific to detox, but if you are aware of any other oils that you would like to use or are currently using other oils, these may be combined in any of the methods prescribed. Please always follow the manufacturer's recommendations.

Juniper

An astringent, antiseptic and detoxifying oil, juniper is often used as a tonic, as it can help to speed up a sluggish circulation and increase elimination of toxins. Juniper is a diuretic – it will relieve the retention of urine – and therefore increases the expulsion of toxins and waste. It speeds up the metabolic rate, which in turn increases the detox rate. As a 'cleansing' oil it works both on a physical and an emotional level – it detoxes both mind and body.

Fennel/sweet fennel

A great oil for the digestion, fennel strengthens peristalsis – the contraction of the intestinal muscles. Fennel is also a diuretic and so prevents water retention. It works as an antiseptic in the urinary tract and kidneys, dealing with any germs and maintaining a favourable environment during detox. Finally, it is a general tonic and helps to increase circulation and remove waste and toxins.

Rosemary

One of the best all-round essential oils, rosemary is a great balancer of moods and physical manifestations. It has a wonderful stimulating effect on the central nervous system and the rest of the body, and is one of the best oils to use as a natural pick-me-up. Rosemary is also a tonic for the heart, skin, kidneys, spleen and blood; it stimulates the circulation and boosts low blood pressure. However, it should not be used by people who have epilepsy.

Lemon grass

A cleansing, refreshing, spicy oil, lemon grass stimulates the digestion and eases any nervous stomach conditions. It promotes the removal of toxins from the body and is antiseptic and bactericidal.

Peppermint

Used as a remedy for digestive problems, peppermint helps the stomach, liver and intestines. It will ease any strain placed on the intestines and stomach during detox, and will decrease swelling and any bloating. Peppermint can also be used to stimulate the mind! Cooling and relaxing, it is often used in stomach pills and in cooling leg or foot balms.

Pine

Best used for inhalations or burning as it is a very strong oil, pine is refreshing, uplifting and stimulating. It has a stimulating effect on the circulation and helps to remove any phlegm or mucus caused by detoxing.

Basil

Stimulating to the brain and uplifting to the mind, basil is used for stomach complaints and can help the digestive system during detox. It boosts confidence and the circulation, and increases low energy. However, it is very potent and should be used sparingly.

Massage

Essential oils should never be applied directly to the skin without first being diluted. This is because they are highly concentrated and can cause irritation or burning in their undiluted state (more than a ton of petals can be required to provide just 2ml of essential oil).

They should be diluted in what are known as carrier oils or base oils – the vegetable or seed oils that we use every day in our kitchens. This may seem a bit crude, but such oils are totally natural and can therefore be absorbed by the skin and act as a moisturiser. Olive, sunflower, safflower, grapeseed, nut and sesame oils are all readily available; macadamia, sweet almond, jojoba and avocado oils are slightly more exotic but can be found in health food stores and some more enlightened chemists.

The ratio of any home-made blend of massage oils should be no more than eight drops of essential oil to every 20ml of carrier or base oil. You should only blend sufficient oils for immediate use – essential oils are a natural preservative, but if stored incorrectly the blend can become stale or rancid.

Take a plastic bottle or bowl and pour in 20ml of base oil. Add your desired essential oil drop by drop and stop when the blend has a sufficiently strong fragrance for your taste – some oils are stronger than others and you may only need two or three drops. Remember, eight drops is the maximum – it is always better to have less essential oil than more, because using too much can sometimes cause headaches.

Use the blend as you would in a normal massage, or follow the self-massage sequence in Chapter 4. When the massage is complete try to keep the oil on your skin for at least an hour, which will allow it to continue being absorbed. If you need to dress after a massage, wipe off any excess oil first because it may colour or stain your clothing.

If you have a ready-made blend you can apply it directly to your skin as a body oil or you can just rub a few drops around your high stomach area (solar plexus) about where the ribs divide. This will be absorbed into your digestive system and will encourage the detox.

Bathing

If you are going to add essential oils to your bath, as with massage, they should never be used before being diluted in base or carrier oils (see above) or a dispersant. The two most readily available dispersants in the average household are milk or high-volume alcohol (vodka is best, as it has no fragrance and no sugar content). These products will break down the essential oil into much smaller droplets, which will make it spread more evenly in the water and be less likely to irritate your skin.

Diluting your essential oil with a base or carrier oil will make your bath more oily. This is great when you can massage the residue of oil into your skin after the bath, but if you are bathing first thing in the morning or if you need to get dressed immediately afterwards a dispersant is more practical, since the oils will be absorbed into the skin almost immediately without leaving any greasy residue.

When bathing in oils you should not use soap, which will destroy their effect. Choose a time when you do not need to wash, such as just before bed or after you have taken a quick shower. Run a bath that is hot enough to stay warm for 15 or 20 minutes but not too hot to be uncomfortable to sit in.

Decide whether to use a carrier oil or a dispersant. In either case you need a only tablespoon of it. Add between two and four drops of essential oil. When the bath is full, let the water go calm and then sprinkle the tablespoon of blended oil over the surface.

Close all the windows so that none of the steam escapes. You might also want to light some candles to create a really relaxing, sensuous experience. Slowly get into the bath, then concentrate on breathing slowly and deeply, inhaling all the vapours from the oil. Allow your skin to soak and absorb all the oils. You should be able to relax totally and unwind. Try to detox your mind!

When you have finished your bath, get out slowly. If you have used a carrier oil, try to smooth all the oil from the surface of the water over your skin. Pat yourself dry, letting as much oil as possible stay on your skin as a natural moisturiser and allowing any residual oil to continue to be absorbed. If you have used a dispersant, there will still be a small amount of oil to massage into your skin. If you need to dress after your bath you should be able to let the oil be absorbed as you would a body cream.

Ideally you should now relax or go straight to bed.

Inhalation

Using essential oils for inhalation is an excellent way to benefit from them immediately, without having to remove any clothing. If you breathe in the vapours from the oils they will enter the olfactory system instantly, so you must take care with the amounts used.

First boil some water and pour it into a large bowl. Add two or three drops of your chosen oil – no dispersants or carriers are required as the oil does not come into direct contact with the skin – and lower your head, covered with a towel or sheet, over the bowl. Inhale slowly through your nose and out through your mouth. You can lower your face closer to the water as you become used to the vapour. Inhaling is an excellent method of dealing with colds and coughs as the effects are immediate and the relief is very welcome. Inhale for about five minutes or until you have had enough, then uncover your head and breathe the cool air.

You can also inhale oils by placing two or three drops on an old handkerchief (the oils may stain) and holding it near your nose or mouth. Don't put the hankie directly on the skin as the oils may irritate it.

Compresses

Sometimes nothing more than a hot water bottle is required for relaxation or to relieve discomfort or pain. Using a compress is the aromatherapy equivalent.

Fill a large bowl with hand-hot water, add a couple of drops of your chosen essential oil and soak a large piece of cotton cloth in it for a couple of minutes. Wring out the cloth and fold it into a compress large enough to cover the area of discomfort. Put two further drops of your oil directly onto the compress (it will spread and dilute into the soaked cotton), then hold the compress on the painful area. Use the compress until it cools down, and if you wish you can repeat the process.

The compress method is ideal for period pains, fever, headaches and so on, as the oil can be applied directly in a soothing, relaxing way. You can of course use the compress for any condition or for any reason. If you get a brief chance to sit down and relax during your busy day, a nice lavender and ylang ylang compress (both are oils for relaxation and rejuvenation) would make your five minutes even more relaxing!

Burners

An oil burner is an excellent way of getting essential oils into the atmosphere so that you can benefit from their therapeutic qualities as you go about your everyday business. NB: Oils should not be used when there are children under five in the room or house.

The choice of burner is quite important as there are many that look quite wonderful but are not very practical. You need one with a bowl big enough to contain 120ml (4 fl oz) of water (the equivalent of a small cup). If the bowl holds much more than this it will take too long to heat the water; if it is much smaller it will have burnt dry, giving a rancid smell, before the candle has gone out.

You need to fill the burner with water, light the candle below and then put four or five drops of your chosen essential oil or oils on the surface of the water. You are unlikely to find you have used too much oil in a burner as the vapour will be distributed throughout the building, but if you start to develop a mild headache simply add more water or blow out the candle.

The alternative is to use dry burners. There are terracotta rings available that fit over a light bulb, or electrically heated porcelain plates. You put a few drops of your chosen oil on the heated surface, and the heat creates the vapour. You can control these by either turning off the power to the porcelain plates or removing the terracotta ring from the light bulb burner.

MASSAGE

Alongside aromatherapy, massage is one of the oldest-known forms of complementary therapy. As with aromatherapy, massage can be done on a particular part of the body (for instance face massage or foot massage) or in total (a massage incorporating every part of the body including the stomach and abdomen).

Traditional massage works by increasing the circulation, which in turn helps the efficient flow of lymph. This has a positive effect on the immune system and keeps the body balanced and healthy. During the Detox Programme any therapy that enhances these functions should be encouraged and enjoyed as much as possible. Muscle conditions such as soreness, spasm and tension are all helped by massage, as the increased blood flow and manipulation techniques help to stretch and tone. There are many other side effects of these benefits – better skin tone, relaxed mind, reduced heart rate and so on.

We tend to think of massage as 'Swedish' or 'therapeutic' or 'holistic'. There is not much difference between these, as all massage strokes derive from three original 'Swedish'-named techniques.

- *Effleurage* Flat hands push flesh from the lower body up towards the head and back down the body. This technique is used to warm the muscles and flesh and to increase the circulation prior to deeper work.

- *Pettrissage* Kneading, wringing and pulling the muscles so that the flesh and muscles are worked against each other or the flesh is pressed against the bone to cause deeper friction. This technique is used to tone the muscles and flesh and to work through any tension or spasm.

- *Tapotement* Quick, invigorating strokes such as hacking (the side of the hand is used to 'chop' the skin); cupping (cupped hands are placed in rapid succession on the skin to 'draw' the blood to the surface); and pummelling (hands clenched in fist shapes and placed with the heel of the palm facing down in rapid succession on the skin to cause a deeper impression on the muscles and so increase circulation).

There are many other types of massage: remedial, sports, tai, Indian head and so on. All of these are very valuable, but for the detox process the traditional aromatherapy and massage techniques are the best.

Massage practitioners will use either oils such as the base or carrier oils described for aromatherapy, or a blend of carrier oils and some basic essential oils. During a massage the client lies on a couch, either naked or in their underwear, partially covered in towels or a blanket to keep warm. The room should be warm and peaceful. All massage strokes should be carried out towards the heart as this helps complete the passage of blood throughout the body and increases the circulation of both blood and lymph.

Initial strokes should be relaxing, warming and smooth and should not cause any pain – there may be discomfort, but not actual pain. Strokes should work in time with your breathing and be of a regular pace. As the treatment progresses and the muscles get warmed the strokes can become more vigorous and more intrusive as the practitioner 'milks' the muscles of any toxins and drains the body of any wastes. Once an area has been warmed, very deep, specific work can be carried out which may feel uncomfortable but will help to sort out deep-seated problems or tense muscle conditions.

Whatever the reason for your massage, it should give you an overall feeling of relaxation and well-being if carried out correctly. You may feel 'worked over', but this should be an invigorating feeling and not an exhausted, painful or bruised feeling.

During detox, massage is wonderful. The lighter strokes relax and warm you, the deeper strokes sort out your muscles and increase the circulation to help the internal cleansing process, and the invigorating strokes stimulate and give you a truly vital feeling. Can you tell that I trained as a massage therapist?

AN IMPORTANT DISTINCTION

A common mistake to make is to think that aromatherapy and massage are the same thing. Aromatherapy massage treatments are designed to facilitate the optimum absorption of the essential oils. The treatment warms the flesh, which increases the circulation so that the body can absorb the oils completely. It is the therapeutic quality of the oils that work and trigger effects within the body while the client receives the treatment, and not the physical treatment itself.

By comparison, massage treatments are designed to improve the body's circulation, lymph flow and immune system entirely through the physical use of different speed, length and pressure of strokes. You will feel much more 'worked' after a massage treatment than you should after an aromatherapy treatment.

Each technique is beneficial in its own right, and clients should be aware of the differences in order to decide which is best for them. A sore back the day after a full afternoon of gardening can be treated by either massage or aromatherapy, but see how the approach varies.

Massage would warm and stretch the muscles so that the tension is soothed and the circulation to the muscles increased to help them work efficiently. A combination of deep friction work and stretching strokes would be recommended. Alternatively, aromatherapy oils such as ginger and black pepper are warming to the muscles, so would be used in combination with long, slow strokes, increasing the blood supply to the surface of the flesh to ensure the optimum absorption of oils. The results would be the same in either case – a fully relaxed body with stretched and relaxed muscles.

REFLEXOLOGY

This technique is based on the principle of reflex points or zones on the feet relating to points, organs and systems within the body. By working with these zones or points the practitioner can treat areas of illness, imbalance or weakness. It is a very old technique, recorded as far back as ancient Egyptian times. Reflexology is an excellent diagnostic tool as it can reveal any problems within the body, even in the early stages. The practitioner can then work on them before any further, more serious conditions develop.

During a reflexology treatment the client sits or lies on a treatment couch while the practitioner follows a sequence around each foot that covers every reflex point or zone. The practitioner will ask the client to identify areas of discomfort or pain, which can then be 'worked' to improve the condition. Reflexology practitioners often use calendula powder or ordinary talc to make the treatment go smoothly.

During the Detox Programme it is likely that your internal systems and organs will be working harder or differently from the way they would normally work. Reflexology can help the body detox by 'balancing' organs like the kidneys and liver, helping the intestines to carry out their cleansing function without causing any unnecessary pressure or imbalance.

Reflexology can also tell you what your body requires or simply what it is going through. If you have treatments while you are detoxing you will often find 'tender points' in the bladder, kidney and digestive system, all of which are working hard. The practitioner will work on these specific points to bring them to optimum condition for continued cleansing.

Reflexology treatments will also show up any potential imbalance, and the practitioner can work at a preventative level. If you are super-healthy or your detox has made your body totally balanced, these treatments are just as useful for maintenance and prevention, and, in any case, they always offer a relaxing, soothing, hour-long treatment.

COLONIC IRRIGATION

Although it has been around since as early as 1500 BC, colonic irrigation seems to be a relatively new and experimental therapy for most people. It consists of an internal 'bath' that helps to cleanse the colon of accumulated poisons, gases, faecal matter and mucus deposits. The practitioner gently pumps filtered water into your rectum, which will start to soften and flush away any build-up of toxins and waste.

Colonic irrigation is extremely effective during the Detox Programme. While you are on the programme you will be eliminating all sources of toxins from your diet, which means that any toxins in your body that are eliminated in waste matter will not be replaced. But there will still be a build-up of toxins within your body from years of 'toxic living'. While foods such as brown rice, nuts and pulses will help to break this down, colonic irrigation will speed up the process and actively flush out the detritus.

The colonics practitioner will ask you to lie on a couch or plinth, with your lower body covered with a towel or sheet. Filtered water, at a carefully regulated temperature, is introduced under gentle gravitational pressure through the rectum and into the colon. The practitioner will use massage to help the water soften and cleanse the colon of faecal matter and waste, which is flushed away with the waste water. The colon is worked on in stages: each time water is pumped in and flushed out, until the colon is completely cleansed. The practitioner will also suggest how many further treatments are required, and recommend appropriate supplements to replace natural bowel fibre and flora. The entire session will last less than an hour.

Practitioners are totally aware of the 'unusual' circumstances in which they have to place their clients, and discretion and modesty are observed throughout. The after-effects of colonic irrigation are similar to those of the entire Detox Programme: a feeling of well-being, lightness, mental clarity and increased energy, a loss of any bloated feeling, relief from constipation and clearer, glowing skin.

Colonics is not something that normally springs to mind as a complementary therapy – people normally think of massage or aromatherapy. But if you have ever thought about trying this treatment to see what the effects would be, or if you believe it might help but have never got round to booking a session, this is the time to try! It's painless, it's different, it makes you feel great and it's detoxifying.

MOISTURISING

During the Detox Programme you will be doing many new and different things to your body, most of which will involve an increased level of activity either internally or externally. During any process the body will be using up fluids in exercise, sweating, cell regeneration, elimination of toxins, cleansing and so on. This fluid must be replaced if your body is to maintain optimum levels of detoxing.

You already know that you need to drink at least 1.5 litres (2³/₄ pints) of water a day to keep your fluid levels steady, but you also need to make sure that other kinds of moisture are topped up. Each time you bath, wash, receive a treatment or carry out any of the body-care treatments essential to the programme, you should moisturise your skin.

Maintaining the skin moisture levels on your body as well as your face is important to detox. Keeping your skin cells and flesh in good condition will help to:

• Give your skin a warm glow.

• Allow your skin to shed old dead cells more effectively.

• Stop your skin looking dry and dull.

A daily skin-care routine is essential if you want it to stay in optimum condition. Remember, it is better to do a little and often (simply wash with water and follow with a moisturiser every day), than to do a lot infrequently (cleanse, tone, scrub, face mask and exfoliate once a month or when you can remember). Despite what the ads would have us believe, creams and gels are not the only way to keep the skin's natural moisture levels – oils are just as effective, if not better.

10

The Only Way to Banish Cellulite

Cellulite is one of the most hotly debated subjects in the health and beauty world. It has been around for ever, but the constant development of many so-called anti-cellulite creams and lotions by the cosmetics industry has given us hope. For a price, we are now led to believe that we can 'reduce the effects of cellulite' or banish it altogether. The truth is that, unless we undergo surgery, the only way to get rid of cellulite or actually to improve the condition is to change what we feed our bodies, how we exercise our bodies and how we treat our bodies, and even then, nothing in this life is guaranteed ...

Most Western women have cellulite because of their lifestyle – our diet and level of activity – rather than as a result of the genes we inherit. So this is something that we can change if we want to. By comparison, Oriental women, with a different lifestyle and different diet, are historically less likely to develop cellulite. That said, the advent and introduction of our 'fast-food outlets' into these countries in the name of progress has started to see a change – we are exporting cellulite! And then there is nature, some cultures are less prone to it than others simply because general body proportions and fat cell distribution vary between the different cultures.

Contrary to popular belief, female hormones don't actually cause cellulite, although they do assist its progress. This helps to explain why it is more likely to develop during puberty, pregnancy and the menopause – times when the hormone balance is disrupted. In the same way, women who take hormone supplements such as the contraceptive pill or HRT will also be altering the body's normal state. This may increase bloating, or the body's ability to process fluids and lymph efficiently, and so increase the possibility of developing cellulite. Similarly, people who are continually yo-yo dieting will also disrupt the body's normal flows and functions.

Unfortunately, however, cellulite doesn't just disappear when hormonal shifts stop. Although our bodies all have the same number of fat cells, hormones determine their size, shape, accumulation and distribution. Stress, a sedentary lifestyle, dress, posture, bad circulation, diet and bingeing all contribute to its formation.

Men also get cellulite. Their hormones programme it to collect above and around their waist, where their fat cells are more concentrated, whereas female hormones programme it to collect on the hips and thighs where fat is concentrated in readiness for childbirth. Cellulite also looks different on men because their connective tissue is firmer and more tightly packed, and because their skin is thicker and has a higher percentage of muscle fibre, 40–45 per cent compared with 30 per cent in women.

When the circulation becomes sluggish, toxins, waste products and slow-moving lymph fluid collects between these connective tissues, resulting in cellulite. Its superficial appearance can vary widely. Some people develop a fairly consistent 'orange peel' effect on their skin, whereas others have irregular lumps, and sometimes cellulite is barely noticeable because that person's skin is so well toned.

So how do we change the factors that we *can* influence? How do we stop the circulation becoming sluggish, and the lymph flow slowing down and collecting between the connective tissue? How do we get rid of all the other lifestyle factors that increase our propensity to develop cellulite? It's a question of bringing the body back into balance and maintaining this state. The answer is quite simple – detox! The Detox Programme is the only truly effective anti-cellulite programme. Diet is addressed, exercise is addressed, posture is addressed, the skin is addressed and all relevant treatments are addressed. So the good news is that if you are on the programme you will inevitably reduce any cellulite you might have – what a side effect!

A CLOSER LOOK AT THE CAUSES

By taking a closer look at the causes of cellulite you will see how the Detox Programme really is the only solution.

Poor eating habits

The downside of convenience foods

If you don't watch what you eat or you eat 'on the hoof', grabbing pre-packed foods or ready meals, it is likely that your diet will be high in fats and sugars. When these are broken down by the metabolism much of the product is surplus to nutritional requirements, and the result is fat. In women this fat naturally accumulates around the thigh and buttock area. Extra weight places a strain on the skin cells and tissue. The constant straining of this tissue will eventually result in permanent weakness, which manifests itself in sagging, drooping flesh. This lack of skin tone is likely to make the cellulite more visible.

Diets and binges: the yo-yo effect

If you continually change the way you eat, one week eating masses of food and the following week next to nothing because you are 'dieting', your body will do everything in its power to reduce this fluctuation – it goes into 'starvation mode'. To regulate the peaks and troughs of diet–binge eating, the metabolism slows down in order not to burn the fat. By doing so, it will have stores of fat to use as energy the next time it is starved. The result is that, even if you 'diet', you don't lose weight. If you start to increase the quantities you eat over a short period of time your body is not ready to deal with the overload – it is not in a position automatically to raise its metabolic rate – and so you feel bloated, your circulation and lymph system are overstretched, and you cannot process the waste and excess efficiently. This results in the waste being stored in the body and increases the occurrence of cellulite.

The perils of an imbalanced diet

If you eat an imbalanced diet you will not be providing your body with the essential nutrients it requires to process food and maintain your body in peak condition. A diet full of ready-made, pre-packed or processed foods is a diet full of colourings, flavourings, preservatives and sweeteners. It is also probably a sodium-dominant diet (see page 228). There may not be enough fibre in the diet, and the fresh-foods content will be almost non-existent. When the body has been fuelled by such sub-standard nutrients over an extended period of time the result will be tiredness and lethargy, muscle aches and fatigue.

Unidentified food intolerances

Personal food intolerances are foods that our bodies find difficult to process. However, we are usually unaware of this and continue to eat these foods, regardless, because we like the taste. Eventually the body compromises and finds a way to deal with the difficult foods in our system in order to function effectively, but this can cost us. For example, we may feel sluggish or tired, we may get headaches or skin complaints, and in some cases, we pay in cellulite.

The most common food intolerances are to:

- All dairy products
- Caffeine
- Alcohol
- Malt
- Nuts
- Yeast

- Wheat-based products (flour, bread, pasta, etc.)
- Barley
- Maize
- Rye
- Refined flours
- Chocolate
- Refined sugar
- Refined starch

Some easy ways to detect intolerances are to identify what you depend on in your diet and what you crave. The foods that you eat a lot of and regularly, such as bread and cheese, may be doing more harm than good and should be reduced or eliminated from your diet.

Also, you may not eat certain foods very often, but they could be causing some unwanted side effects. Pay attention to any recurrent symptoms, such as headaches, for example, and see if you can associate them with a certain food. I started to notice that, occasionally, when I finished my meal, I started to sound as if I had a bad cold. It turned out that I was finishing with a cheese plate each time it was happening, so I realised I was cheese-intolerant. It was a huge relief, as initially I thought I might be intolerant to red wine!

The sodium–potassium imbalance

The careful balance of sodium and potassium in our bodies is crucial to the efficient flow of oxygen, essential nutrients and waste to and from our cells. Sodium is found mainly inside the cells and potassium outside the cells. Essentially the sodium–potassium balance within the body creates a fully functioning 'pump' – sodium absorbs and potassium expels. If this pump is imbalanced and the sodium is allowed to become dominant, movement between cells becomes sluggish, the removal of waste slows down and leads to build-up, fluid is retained and congestion occurs. The short-term effects are bloating and fluid retention, the long-term ones bad cell renewal and regeneration, which damages the internal structure of the cells.

Our diet can become dominated by salt, which is predominantly sodium chloride. All processed foods contain added salt; we typically add salt to our food as we are cooking it and then add more on the plate when we sit down to eat. Our taste buds can become so used to salt that we gradually increase our tolerance, and in turn our intake.

It is very difficult, on a day-to-day basis, to include enough potassium in your diet to balance the high levels of additional sodium, as it would need to contain twice as much potassium as sodium in order to create a healthy flow of nutrients and expel waste efficiently. There are a number ways in which you can reduce the sodium–potassium imbalance:

- Avoid processed, canned and ready-made foods.

- Never add salt when cooking and reduce the amount of salt you put on your plate. Taste the food first and then add salt only in small amounts. (We automatically tend to add salt without first giving the taste of the food a chance.)

- If your food seems short on flavour look to other seasonings and herbs for an alternative: cayenne pepper, black or white pepper, garlic, and so on, will all add flavour and possibly introduce a new taste experience as well as extra nutrients.

- Canned fish often comes in brine, which is salt water. Canned vegetables come in water with added salt. If you rinse these before eating them you will dramatically reduce your salt intake.

- Beware the word 'sodium' in an ingredient – it means salt. Always read the list of ingredients on packaged foods (bicarbonate of soda is sodium bicarbonate; monosodium glutamate, sodium sulphite and sodium benzoate are all commonly found).

- Increase your intake of potassium-rich foods such as potatoes, melon, carrots, broccoli, papaya, watermelon, Brussels sprouts, sprouted beans and sprouted seeds and all other fresh vegetables.

- Eat more beans (kidney beans, black beans, aduki beans, and so on).

- Eat your vegetables raw. Alternatively, cook them in the smallest possible amount of water or steam them lightly. Better still, use the liquid you cooked the vegetables in to make soup or stock.

STRESS

You may not easily make the connection between stress and cellulite, and it is even more unlikely that you will make the connection between stress and the sodium–potassium balance in the body. But there most certainly is a connection, and it goes like this. Stressful situations trigger a release of the hormone adrenaline to various parts of the body – legs to run away, shoulders and arms to fight and so on. This is the fight-or-flight response that was referred to earlier. Adrenaline also affects many other functions, including water regulation. Increased stress levels cause increased release of adrenaline, which causes imbalance in sodium–potassium levels, which causes bloating and fluid retention.

Stress is also a self-perpetuating condition. We are stressed and we get tired. We do not or cannot do anything about reducing the stress. This becomes stressful in itself and we become even more stressed (and so on and so on).

If you are under stress you should try to look at the causes and then make some changes that will alleviate or remove the triggers. In the meantime you can introduce some simple tools into your life that will have many benefits:

• Drink water to stay hydrated 1.5 litres (2³/₄ pints)

• A balanced, healthy diet

• Breathing techniques

• Relaxation technique

- Exercise

- Affirmations

- Positive thinking

- Massage

- Aromatherapy

- Relaxation

- Walking

All these subjects are covered in depth in Chapters 4 and 9.

POSTURE AND CLOTHING

The importance of good posture

The body is designed with sufficient spacing for our internal organs and systems to function correctly and without hindrance. Changing this spacing through bad posture means the body has to operate in an unnatural and forced environment. Restricted blood flow, inability to breathe deeply, squashed flesh, restricted stomach movement and muscle shortening cause inefficient flow of blood, lymph and waste within the body. The result is congestion, which leads to cellulite.

Avoid restrictive clothing

Another way in which we destroy this spacing is by wearing restrictive clothing. The current fashion for 'skinny' jeans is nothing new; I well remember the fashion for purchasing a tight pair of jeans and then wearing them in the bath to shrink them even further, until the only way to get them done up was to use a hook to pull up the zip while wriggling on the floor. It seems we are right back there, but now, at least, they are pre-shrunk to avoid the pneumonia. I also remember the wide belts that pulled in your waist until breathing became an optional extra. Well, they seem to be back in as well. Remember teetering on four-inch heels as an adolescent to try to gain those all-important inches? Yep, they're back as well. All these 'fashions' (and they will be back around again before we know it – so throw nothing out – unless, of course, you are detoxing your space) restrict not only normal day-to-day physical movement but also natural movement within the body. This restriction results in congestion and so increases the likelihood of cellulite.

INACTIVITY

In any one day we typically spend eight hours lying down and eight hours sitting down. The remainder is split between standing and walking. We lie down to sleep, we sit in a car, we sit on the bus, we sit on the train, we sit at a desk, we sit watching a movie, we sit watching television, we sit down to eat, we stand talking to colleagues or neighbours, we sit with young children while they are going to sleep, we sit down to rest.

We know that mobility is important in old or ill people in order to prevent muscle wastage, bed sores, weakness, oedema, bad circulation and poor respiration, but we never stop to think that any of these might happen to us. If they did it would be an extreme case, but if we don't take care, our ankles can become swollen or our circulation sluggish just through living normally.

Make a note of your daily activity levels. How much time do you spend sitting down? How often do you take the car when you could walk? How often does your leisure activity include sitting or standing still? Change just one of these each day and you will notice the effects on your circulation almost immediately. Good circulation means efficient processing and elimination of waste products which in turn eliminates cellulite. Try:

- Stretching

- Exercise

- Movement of all kinds

- Cold-water splashing

- Cold showers

- Saunas

Make sure you get some exercise every day. It will increase your muscle tone, which will improve the appearance of your body; it also increases circulation and lymph flow. Dry-skin brushing (see page 74) is an excellent means of 'kick-starting' the circulation first thing in the morning and last thing at night. The muscle action required to skin-brush is quite vigorous in itself, but the main benefits are found in the sloughing off of dead cells, which allows the skin to breathe more efficiently, and the boost to circulation from the brushing itself. Anything you can do to extend and contract the muscles in your body will help keep your circulation, skin tone and condition in tip-top order.

ANTI-CELLULITE CHECKLIST

The checklist below will ensure that you follow an anti-cellulite programme. All the areas are covered in depth elsewhere in the book, but this list will act as an aide-memoire towards your cellulite-free future.

- Eat fresh fruit every day.

- Eat fresh vegetables every day.

- Eat rice, beans and pulses every day.

- Eat oily fish regularly.

- Where possible buy organic foods.

- If you change from a diet of mainly processed foods, invest in a good vitamin supplement – multivitamins with no added yeast, flour or talcum.

- Avoid drugs, prescribed or other. Ask your doctor for possible alternatives.

- Avoid hormone pills.

- Eliminate processed foods.

- Eliminate pre-packed foods.

- Eliminate ready-made meals.

- Drink at least 1.5 litres (2³/₄ pints) of water a day.

- Drink herbal teas or hot water with lemon and honey.

- Limit your dairy foods or eliminate them altogether.

- Reduce your fat intake.

- Reduce your sugar intake.

- Reduce your salt intake.

- Do more exercise.

- Adjust your posture – don't cross your legs!

- Don't sit down!

- Reduce any stress in your life and avoid stressful situations – try without becoming stressed about it.

- Dry-skin brush every morning.

- Dry-skin brush every evening.

- Self-massage every morning.

- Self-massage every evening.

- Cold shower or cold bath every day.

- Moisturise your skin every day.

- Breathe deeply.

- Smile, inwardly and outwardly!

Useful Addresses

Contact the appropriate organisation for names of fully qualified, registered practitioners in your local area.

Institute for Complementary Medicine
British Register of Complementary Therapists
PO Box 194
London SE16 1QZ
Tel: 0207 237 5165
Fax: 0207 237 5175
www.i-c-m.org.uk
info@i-c-m.org.uk

For Jane Scrivner Detox salons, spas and practitioners go to:
www.janescrivner.com
info@janescrivner.com

Index